Intermittent fasting for women over 50

start a healthy weight loss lifestyle with this cookbook and detoxify your body, increasing longevity & energy. Enjoy a new fit life with tasty recipes.

Rihanna Johnson

Table of Contents

INTRODUCTION

Thank you for buying this book, and congratulations on making the decision to change your life. The chapters of this book were created to examine all that is necessary to understand to begin intermittent fasting. It is a fantastic diet strategy that focuses more on the right time to eat food instead of the actual foods you are eating. When it comes to using Fast Newspaper to have the ability to make it work for your lifestyle, there is a wide range of alternatives. This overview will provide you with all the information you need to get started with Intermittent Fast. We will see what this fast is about, the health benefits that are included, how to eat with this method of diet, and much more. We will also respond to some typical fasting concerns to make sure you are well prepared to begin. Intermittent fasting can be an exceptional alternative for those who may have problems losing weight in the past and want something that works well for them now. Be sure to consult this manual to begin intermittent fasting today. There are many offers of publications on this subject in the market, so thanks again for choosing this. Each initiative was taken aims to ensure that it is well packaged and full of useful information. So take your time and enjoy it!

Challenges with the modern diet

According to a study by Psychology Today Food and Wellness, 52 percent of Americans believe they find it much less complicated to learn taxes than to know how to eat healthy and balanced foods. Many people have difficulties with the current tax code, which indicates that many more people have trouble discovering exactly how to consume a diet that is exceptional for them. We all understand that we should eat healthier foods. We are also aware that we must precisely limit the number of soft drinks, fruit juices, processed foods and sugars we consume. Although we understand these things, this does not mean that it is so easy to follow. We live in a nation that has difficulties with weight problems. Two out of three adults are related as obese or overweight. Many elements increase weight problems. There has been a unanimous decrease in the quality of our dietary regimes as we move from a country that depends on regional agricultural food to a country where most of our food is mass produced. Since it is often conveniently offered today, this change has improved our food consumption.

Many easy-to-eat and straightforward foods are rich in fat, sugar, and calories. From the desserts, to all the junk food chains that surround us, the quality of the food, and the amount we eat has changed significantly. The first aspect we should observe is the amount of food we consume. The variety of calories that each person requires differs from one person to another. The reference specification used on food labels is around 2000 calories per day. Also, it is easily possible to consume 2000 calories or more.

While eating in restaurants often takes us beyond the calorie limits, it is also possible to consume more even when we consume at home. It is essential to discover how to start drinking what we need, instead of eating because something has an exceptional taste. To identify the typical amount of daily calories ingested by American organizations, look at the amount of food readily available to an individual as an indicator of the amount of food consumed. When considering that some of these foods are wasted or thrown away every day instead of being consumed, the average American still consumes 2700 calories per day. Now, we have to talk about the high quality of the foods that different Americans eat. As we mature, many of us learn from our parents and teachers which foods are appropriate and which are not. Fruits and vegetables are considered fantastic, and sweets and sugars are not. Since they were excellent in small quantities, the rest of the foods may not have been so useful to you even though we were educated about healthy and healthy eating at an early age; it is much harder to follow this guide. According to a survey conducted by the United States Department of Agriculture, in the United States, the six primary sources of calories for most Americans are cereal desserts, yeast bread, poultry, soda/sports drinks, as well as energy and alcoholic drinks. From this main list of five, most of the foods that Americans eat are improved sugars and cereals. According to a research study conducted by the United States Department of Agriculture (USDA) in 2010, eggs, meat, and nuts represent 21% of these diets; oils and fats are 23%, while caloric sugar is 15%. Foods that are not so excellent for us constitute a substantial 61 percent of our dietary strategies. The time of day we consume may also be important. Most Americans live an almost active lifestyle and do not have time to sit and eat a healthy meal. Instead, they eat on the go, usually in a harmful place, or when their metabolic process is slower, they consume at night. Many Americans relax on the couch and also consume unhealthy snacks while watching television. Occasionally, food is so abundant that we eat continuously. It is necessary to identify the activities required to limit the amount of food we eat daily. It is tempting to eat foods that are offered quickly. However, if you want to regain your health and well-being and also stay in good shape, it is essential to stay away from the standard American diet and also choose something healthier and better for you. When you hear about not eating due to religious elements, you can think of people who spend weeks without food. You can feel that it is harmful, or you won't have the chance to do it because you love the excess food. However, recurring fasting differs from spiritual fasting, although they share some common ideas. Recurring concerns about fasting limit calorie intake during some parts of the day or, if not, eat on specific days. Your body still receives the nutrients it needs, but you eat fewer calories for this reason, which facilitates weight loss. The various forms of intermittent fasting will be discussed later in the guide. The reason why this dietary strategy is useful is that it works to reduce the amount of fat left in your body, in addition to the variety of calories you are eating. Since the time allowed to eat or reduce calorie intake during the week is decreasing, it is much easier to minimize the number of calories in general. You can also choose the period in which you wish to participate in the periodic fast. Some classifications of people choose to do it for a month or even more, while others adapt it to their lifestyle, so it becomes long term.

Meaning of intermittent fasting

Since we take time to see how the American diet makes us undesirable, let's look at a diet that will make it easier to lose weight and be healthier. This area of this book will discuss what intermittent fasting is all about, so you can understand how it might work for you.

Intermittent fasting includes a cyclic diet between the periods in which they are allowed to eat, as well as the periods in which they are expected to fast. If you want to lose weight or have much better health, it is much better to eat balanced foods that benefit you. Intermittent fasting involves limiting the use of food for a certain period and does not include any alteration of the actual food you eat. Intermittent fasting could be considered a natural food model that people also try to apply. It goes back to our ancestors, Paleolithic hunter-gatherers. The current version of an organized program of intermittent fasting can help improve much of health from longevity and aging to body structure, and intermittent fasting for beginners has two policies to follow: (1) Requests for fasting are satisfactory, and they are NOT difficult. (2) Fasting is not rigid; it can be comfortable. From the point of view of a fasting expert, I have some tips for beginners about recurring fasting. There are two important factors for people who prefer intermittent fasting (IF): weight loss or health or both. However, it is excellent to observe these two solutions: more regulations = more difficult = low chance of success; fewer rules = less complicated = high probability of success. When it comes to health and wellness, a 24-hour rest period is healthy, helping to reduce calories without compromising what you like to eat and drink during the day without fasting. Perhaps it will also stimulate your body to create more hormonal growth agents. Yes, this is a hormonal representative of healthy development, just like what is heard in the stars asking to "stay young." The hormonal growth agent has many advantages against aging, and one of the most interesting is fat burning. There are numerous types of intermittent fasting techniques. However, all divide the day or week into periods of consumption and periods of fasting. Without a doubt, this would be considered as a kind of intermittent fasting. With this technique, technically fast for sixteen hours a day and then, eat for eight hours a day.

This form of fasting is also called method 16/8; it is among the pending selections when referring to intermittent fasting. Despite what you may think now, intermittent fasting is less complicated than you think. It does not require much preparation work, and many people who have participated in this diet plan report that they feel better and also have extra power when they start quickly. At first, you may be a little hungry. Do not go very long before the body adapts and gets used to it. The main point to keep in mind is that when you continue on an empty stomach, you are not allowed to eat. However, you can still drink drinks to stay hydrated. Some of the selections consist of tea, coffee, water, and other drinks without calories. Some of these rapids will allow you to eat during periods of fasting, but many will not. Also, it is generally excellent to take a supplement while fasting, as long as it does not contain calories.

How intermittent fasting works

What is intermittent fasting? One thing you should know about intermittent fasting is that you cannot consider it as a diet plan. It is a food model, which requires meal planning to maximize its positive effects on fitness and health. The scheme involves a cycle consisting of separate periods of feeding and fasting. This food model does not require you to change the foods you eat. What you need to change is your eating plan. Now, you may wonder if it is worth making some changes when you should eat. The answer is a resounding, yes. IF is an incredible solution if you want to be slim and stay that way without having to follow crazy and stressful diet plans or concentrate too much on counting calories.

In most cases, this eating pattern also requires maintaining calorie intake. It is an excellent way to preserve muscle mass while maintaining a slim body. It is also the simplest strategy if you want to eliminate unwanted weight and make sure you stay within your goal. You can do it without making excessive changes in your behavior. This makes intermittent fasting simple and feasible, in the sense that anyone can easily do it while it is significant since it creates a positive difference in their weight and health.

How does it work

Our body can handle prolonged periods of not eating. Human bodies have the natural ability to transition between the state of hunger and the state of being fed. When we do not eat for an extended period, the processes that enter our body change. When we eat, our body begins to work to digest it and store the energy received through food. When we are hungry, our body begins to take energy from those stored fats. When we are fasting for a certain time, our blood sugar and insulin levels experience a decrease in their levels. It is normal because it pushes our bodies to prosper from the existing resources present in our bodies. Research has shown that fasting helps protect against diseases such as heart disease, diabetes, cancer, and Alzheimer's disease. Therefore, when you fast, you should not worry about compromising your health. To understand how intermittent fasting works, you must first understand two states. The two states are the fed state and the fast state. By understanding these states, we come to know that our bodies continue to function well, regardless of whether our stomachs are empty or full. By fasting in the state of fed, the body is undergoing a process of digestion and absorption of food. The state begins when you start eating and can last up to three to five hours later. In a fed state, your body shows high levels of insulin, and this acts as a signal for your body to store excessive amounts of calories. This deposit occurs in fat cells. During the period with high insulin levels, the fat burning process stops, and the body switches to glucose consumption since its last meal. Then comes a state called post-absorption, which lasts approximately 8-12 hours after the last meal. Subsequently, the body enters a state of fasting. In a state of fasting; The body does not process any food, and insulin levels are low. This induces the mobilization of stored body fat that resides within the body in fat cells and begins to burn these fats to provide energy to the body. In this state, the body can burn fat that was previously inaccessible during the fed state. Staying hungry for a certain period helps you with hundreds of things. When you eat a meal, your body is in a "fed state" and processes only the food you just ate. After a few hours and the food is completely digested, you go to an intermediate stage where you are not hungry but have not eaten anything else. You can call it an intermediate state. Eight to twelve hours after the last meal, when you are hungry and fasting, a state called "fasting state" appears. In this state, your body needs to recover fuel to function, but it cannot find energy. Then, it starts looking for energy sources inside the body. It starts by going to the fat cells where the fats from your previous meals were stored. The body is designed to store a certain amount of fat from each meal to recover energy when necessary. Therefore, due to low insulin levels, the body has now entered a state of fat burning and begins to burn the fats present in the body. This is useful in hundreds of ways. Not only will it eliminate excess fat from you, but it will also eliminate all the toxins present inside the body.

Toxins can be anything harmful present in your body. It can be a dysfunctional cell or a cell that is damaged and does not work well. The removal of these cells is very necessary when we talk about maintaining health. Therefore, it is necessary to be in a "fasting state" so that the body can initialize the combustion state. Intermittent fasting offers you a convenient way to fast and eliminate excess fat, calories, and damaged cells. Many health professionals and doctors recommend them.

Patients start fasting for this purpose. They believe that health will improve if they fast because of this quality of intermittent fasting.

How is intermittent fasting more risky for women?

Women who participate in studies around the world and those who report their results on social networks or in fitness communities report many of the same negative effects that men experience during the process of adapting to a new fasting plan. Some of these side effects include:

• Initial hunger and dehydration pains

• Difficulty concentrating or increasing concentration during the day

• Headache, muscle weakness, the initial loss of muscle tone There are some effects that women have experienced and should be observed, especially those with a history of problems or concerns with their menstrual cycles. One of these reported negative effects is infertility after long periods in an intermittent fasting plan. This tends to happen more in women who experience a dramatic loss of body fat, especially in the first weeks (or during the period of adaptation).

• In most women, this is not a permanent problem, as periods generally return to normal and fertility increases in the weeks following the interruption of an intermittent fasting plan, particularly for reasons of weight loss.

• Most health experts and medical professionals recommend pregnant women, or those who expect to become pregnant shortly, avoid starting or suspending your intermittent fasting plan before making sure they are fit. They minimize their chances of conceiving. However, for those interested in starting an intermittent fast, it is important to keep in mind that although fasting is still studied worldwide for its long term benefits, it risks almost everyone who might be interested in it (age, sex, contests, cultural diets, health stories). Health and wellness experts from around the world have written and talked about its safety, its benefits, and its promising progress, for men and women. It all comes down to being prepared, having all the right information, and making a plan that works and can be maintained in the long term.

Advantages of intermittent fasting

Intermittent fasting has incredible benefits not only for the body and brain of women but also for men. The following are some of the benefits related to intermittent hunger:

It alters the functioning of the body's cells and hormones: intermittent fasting practiced for a while brings several changes in your body. For your body to produce more accessible fats, it tends to initiate important cellular repair processes and also changes the hormonal levels in your body. Insulin levels in your body decrease by facilitating the breakdown of fats. Growth hormones also increase when blood levels increase a factor that facilitates muscle gain. The body induces processes such as cell repair and the elimination of any waste material from cells.

Weight loss and belly calories: intermittent fasting is done to lose weight since you only eat a few meals. Intermittent fasting improves the metabolic rate, which helps the body burn excess fat, such as belly fat. Studies show that intermittent fasting leads to a weight loss of 3-8 percent when performed for approximately three to twenty-four weeks. The observation shows that during this fasting period, 4-7 percent of people have lost abdominal fat, one of the toxic fats in the human body responsible for various diseases. It reduces insulin resistance; intermittent fasting reduces insulin levels in the body, which in turn reduces the risks of type 2 diabetes, which is a common disease. Common features of diabetes include high blood sugar levels in insulin. Therefore, intermittent fasting helps reduce insulin levels, which helps prevent this disease. It also helps protect possible damage that can affect the kidneys. Reduction of constant oxidative worry and inflammation of the body; intermittent fasting helps reduce stress, which is one of the riskiest forms of rapid aging and other chronic diseases. Free radicals are the molecules responsible for the reaction with molecules such as DNA and proteins and their destruction. Intermittent fasting, therefore, helps fight inflammation in the body and destroys the molecules responsible for constant worry.

Heart health: intermittent fasting is beneficial to the health of your heart and prevents you from getting any heart disease. Because it regulates sugar levels in the body, intermittent fasting prevents you from having hypertension, inflammatory markers, and cholesterol levels, thus maintaining heart health. Induction of cell restoration procedures: when you fast, your body begins the "waste disposal" procedures of the cell known as autophagy.

Body cells

The dysfunctional proteins that accumulate within cells of the body are decomposed and metabolized. The increase in waste disposal prevents your body against other diseases such as Alzheimer's disease, one of the common neurodegenerative disorders without treatment.

Cancer prevention: After the body has eliminated dysfunctional cells that accumulate over time, the body is free of any cancer risk. Uncontrolled cell development is one of the common characteristics of cancer and, therefore, intermittent fasting facilitates the body's metabolic rate, which helps reduce potential cancer risks. Intermittent fasting also reduces several impacts of chemotherapy.

Brain health: since intermittent fasting is better for your body, then it is better for your brain. The reduction of oxidative stress and various concerns is beneficial to the physical capacity of the brain. Recurring fasting increases the development of new nerves, improving the functioning of the brain. It also helps increase levels of brain hormones known as brain-derived neurotrophic factors, which help fight depression and any other brain-related disease. Intermittent fasting also helps fight brain damage caused by a stroke.

Prolonged lifespan: intermittent fasting can help you live longer thanks to its ability to control metabolism rates, regulate blood sugar levels, and eliminate dysfunctional cells within your body.

Disadvantages of intermittent fasting

Unfortunately, intermittent fasting also has cons, especially for women. Studies show that before attempting intermittent fasting, you should always contact your doctor. The following are the disadvantages associated with intermittent fasting:

It is not without risks: intermittent fasting is not recommended for people who have greater health risks, such as people over sixty-five. People with medical conditions, high-fat requirements, diabetics, low weight, minors, pregnant women, and babies cannot perform intermittent fasting.

You will be hungry: during intermittent fasting, you may have a stomach ache, especially if you have followed the correct diet plans. You should avoid looking, smelling, or even thinking about food during fasting, as this causes the release of gastric acids in the stomach, which makes you hungry. Participate in other activities, but if you want to fill your water, drink infusions or other non-caloric drinks. You may notice an increase in food consumption on days without eating, where you are not limited to any calorie intake. Intermittent fasting causes excessive food consumption. There may also be cases of birthmarks, especially after the increase in cortisol hormone levels.

Dehydration: lack of food can make you forget to drink water. You cannot take note of the signs of thirst when you fast.

Tiredness: intermittent fasting makes you feel tired, especially if you try for the first time. Your body tends to run out of energy and disrupts your sleep patterns, and this is accompanied by a feeling of tiredness.

Irritability: since intermittent fasting helps regulate mood, it can also regulate appetite. It leads to being depressed and upset.

The long-term consequences of intermittent fasting are unknown: since no one knows if after losing weight, it will remain the same for a few years, studies say there is no relevant evidence to support the extent of intermittent fasting. Therefore, it is always recommended to speak with your doctor for solid advice on how to practice intermittent fasting. Precautions should be taken during intermittent fasting. Fasting has existed since time immemorial, and in some religions, it is considered a sacred practice. Either way, you can start practicing intermittent fasting; it is necessary to follow their essential advice to avoid inconvenience. Therefore, it is necessary:

Make sure your body is fit to fast. Make sure you are not pregnant, not undergoing any treatment, have no health complications, are not a minor, or even diabetic. If you cannot fast, you can always switch to cleaner eating habits, such as eating natural foods and eliminating sugars, rich or fatty foods from your diet. Before beginning intermittent fasting, you should always try to consult your doctor. Your doctor will provide updates on your health problems and advise you if the transition is necessary or not.

Try to adopt intermittent fasting to your lifestyle. You should never fast when you are under excessive stress. If you are a beginner in intermittent fasting, it is advisable to try the 5:2 fast module, where you can fast on the first day of the week and then on Thursday to prepare for your favorite meals on weekends. Before beginning intermittent fasting, do not snuggle up with a "last supper," but you should eat healthy meals, lean proteins, and vegetables. Fruit has natural sugar, and including it in your food could mean a lot. A small amount of starch could also complete the meal. A meal that contains all these nutrients will make your body survive the fasting period.

Prepare your home, body, and thoughts before beginning intermittent fasting. It means you should get enough rest and prepare emotionally. Think about your goal and how to achieve it. Be sure to hide or stay out of reach of any food that may tempt you during the fasting period. Stop pretending to be a hero, even when your body is weak. Do not press your body too much in the name of fasting. Here are some of the symptoms that should be of great concern during fasting: Cardiac tremors, dizziness, and general weakness should be considered. It requires the use of common sense because you cannot force your body to do what it cannot. Do not participate in difficult exercises; make them light. Participate in massages because they help the blood flow in the body parts to be full of calories, reducing cortisol. Do not burn your muscles for energy during fasting.

Always take your vitamins depending on the fasting method you choose. This acts as a supplement, especially in liquid form, as it facilitates the process of digestion. They help compensate for vitamins lost during fasting. Do not forget to drink a lot of water every day while fasting. Urine should warn you if it is not light in color. If it is too dark, drink desirable amounts of water for proper hydration. During fasting, it is an obstacle to associate with your friends while having fun; they are eating chocolates and drinking wine, so you'll be tempted to join them. You can enjoy other ways of having fun with your friends. You can visit the nearest mall, buy new clothes or buy electronic products. Avoid grocery stores and dinner dates. Remove the photos from your gallery that will make your mouth water.

Avoid stress because stress increases cortisol levels, responsible for fat accumulation and muscle breakdown. You can practice yoga, meditate, or breathe deeply. Your body needs enough energy to last during the fasting period, so these exercises should be light and non-vigorous. To avoid going crazy, you can always invite your friends to accompany you on an intermittent fast. An online search for other people performing intermittent fasting can help you track your progress. This is when you should concentrate on mentally cleaning your closet and thinking about what you are doing.

Avoid the "wave of victory." Many people are happy after the fasting period. You should eat a meal and avoid healthy foods that you can easily digest. You should eat foods rich in fiber and, if you are an alcoholic, remember to be careful when drinking.

Types of intermittent fasting

There are so many different ways to practice intermittent fasting that the entire chapter is dedicated only to these methods. I will guide you through 10 specific and different methods for IF before finishing with a section on how to make your choice. At the end of this chapter, if you have chosen to test the IF, you should feel that your IF plans have direction and form, and you should be excited to implement these new plans in your daily routine.

Explanation of different methods.

Before you can start intermittent fasting and incorporate it into your lifestyle, you must know all the possibilities to choose the right one for you, your goals, your habits, and your body/personality type. Read the following ten tips to discover which methods seem most appropriate.

Lean gain method

The method of lean gain essentially focuses on the combined efforts of rigorous exercise, fasting, and a healthy diet. The fame surrounding this approach comes from its acclaimed success in converting fat directly into the muscle. The goal is to fast every day for 14-16 hours, starting from the waking up. The ideal approach to lean gains seems to be to get up and fast until 1:00 pm, stretch, and warm-up before training just before noon. Starting at noon, you would start training in any exercise you choos for an hour or less, and you will end up breaking quickly around 1 pm. Your meal at this time would be the best of the day. You attended your days as always in the past and, as far as possible, return to eat around 4 pm, then eat for the last time around 9 pm. If you choose this approach and feel a little overwhelmed, you can work up to 15 hours, starting with 13 or 14 hours of fasting only during the first week.

Method 16:8

The 16:8 method is one of the most popular among the fasters. You spend 16 hours on an empty stomach every day, and the other 8 hours are your window to eat. Many people try to choose the 8-hour feeding period as the time when they are most active. If you are a night person, do not hesitate to do it a little later. Stop eating during the day as much as possible and then have breakfast around 3 or 4 in the afternoon. For people who have breakfast early in the morning, for example, around 11 am, or lunch from 7 pm to 4 a.m. It is an incredibly flexible method that works for many different types of people. It is also flexible when you decide to try a particular fast food relationship. For example, if you don't seem to be playing with the food window from 11 a.m. to 7 p.m., you can change the next day to meet your needs better. You can try to wait until later for breakfast! Try what you need to do, as long as you keep that ratio of 16:8 hours. While the lean gain method technically applies the same hourly rate, it is much more rigorous than a healthy diet and exercise regime. The 16:8 method does not need any exercise reinforcement, but it depends on the professional. It is always better to try to add healthy dietary options to your IF feeding schedule, but do not try to limit too many calories, as it may cause dizziness and low energy. With 16:8, you can eat what you need and exchange the hoursyouwant.

Method 14:10

Similar to method 16:8, 14:10 requires fasting and feeding on multiple levels every day. In this case, I would fast for 14 hours and then eat for 10 hours. This method has the same flexibility of 16:8 in terms of what time of day it is organized and how easy it is to solve problems. But it is also flexible in the sense that the window for eating lasts two hours longer, it can accommodate people with more intense physical routines or daily needs, as well as people who need to eat a little later during the day.

Method 20:4

While the 14:10 method was a simpler step than the 16:8 method, the 20:4 method is a step forward in terms of difficulty. Without a doubt, it is a more intense method, since it requires 20 hours of fasting every day with only a 4-hour feeding period for the individual to obtain all their nutrients and energy. Many people who try this method end up eating a large meal with several snacks or two smaller meals with fewer snacks. The 20:4 method is flexible in the sense where the individual chooses how the window for eating is divided between meals and snacks.

The 20:4 method is complicated since many people instinctively eat excessively during the feeding window, but it is neither necessary nor healthy. People who choose the 20:4 method should try to keep portions of food the same size they normally would without fasting. Experiencing how many snacks are needed will also be useful in this method. Many people end up working up to 20:4 with other methods, depending on what their bodies are capable of handling and what they are ready to try. Few begin with 20:4, so if it doesn't work right away, don't be too hard on yourself! Return to 16:8 and then see how soon you can return to where you want to be.

The warrior method

The warrior's method is quite similar to the 20:4 method in which the individual fasts for 20 hours a day and stops quickly for a period of 4 hours to eat. However, the difference lies in the perspective and mentality of the professional. The thought process behind the warrior's method is that in ancient times, the hunter who returned home from stalking prey or the warrior who returned home from the battle only received one meal a day. A meal should provide sustenance for the rest of the day, recovering energy for the future. Therefore, warrior method professionals are advised to eat an excellent meal when they have breakfast and that the meal should be rich in fat, protein, and carbohydrates for the rest of the day (and for the days to come). However, as with the 20:4 method, it can sometimes be too intense for professionals, and it is very easy to reduce it a lot by inventing a method like 18:6 or 17:7. If it doesn't work, don't force it, but try to do it for a week to see if the problem is your stubbornness or if it is just a coincidence with the method.

12:12 Method

The 12:12 method is somewhat simpler, along with the lines of 14:10, instead of 16:8 or 20:4. Beginners in intermittent fasting would do well to try immediately. Some people sleep 12 hours every night and can easily wake up from the fasting period, ready to join the window to eat. Many people use this method in their lives without even knowing it. However, to follow the 12:12 method in your life, you will want to be as determined as possible. Be sure to be strict with the limits of 12 hours. Make sure it works and feels good in your body, so we invite you to improve things and try, for example, 14:10 or maybe your invention, like 15:11. As always, start with what works and then go up (or down) to what makes you feel good (and maybe even better).

5:2 method

The 5:2 method is popular among those who wish to improve things in general. Instead of fasting and eating every day, these people practice fasting two full days a week. The other five days are free to eat, exercise or diet, but the other two days (which can be consecutive or scattered during the week) must be strictly fasting days. However, for those fasting days, it is not as if the individual can not eat anything at all. It is allowed to consume no more than 500 calories per day for this intermittent fasting method. I suppose that these days of fasting would be better known as "limited hiring" days, as it is a more precise description. The 5:2 method is extremely rewarding, but it is also one of the most difficult to try. If you have problems with this method, do not be afraid to experiment next week with a method like 14:10 or 16:8, where you fast and eat every day. If this works best for you, stick with it! However, if you have "active" days and "free" days with fasting and feeding, there are also other alternatives.

Eat-Stop-Eat method (24 hours)

The method to stop eating for 24 hours is another option for people who want to have "on" and "free" days between fasting and eating. It is a little less intense than the 5:2 method and is much more flexible for the individual, depending on what he needs. For example, if you need a 24-hour literal fast every week and that's it, you can do it. On the other hand, if you want something more flexible than the type of 5:2 method to happen, you can work with what you want and create a method that surrounds those desires and goals. The most successful approaches to the Eat-Stop-Eat method involved a more rigorous diet (or at least a prudent and healthy diet) during the 5 or 6 days in which the individual participates in the free meal window of the week. For the individual to see success with weight loss, there will also have to be a caloric restriction (or a high nutrition approach) those 5 or 6 days, so that the body has a version of consistency in the health content, and nutrition. In the one or two days a week that the individual decides to fast, there may still be a very limited calorie intake. As with the 5:2 method, during these fasting days, you cannot consume more than 500 calories in food and beverages so that the body can maintain the flow of energy and more.

If the individual exercises, those training days must be reserved for 5 or 6 days of free food. The same applies to method 5:2. Try not to exercise (at least not in excess) on the days chosen to fast. Your body will not appreciate the additional stress when you eat so few calories. As always, you can choose to switch from Eat-Stop-Eat to another method if it works easily, and you are interested in something else. Also, you can start with a rigorous 24-hour method and then move on to a more flexible Eat-Stop-Eat approach. Do what you think is right and never be afraid to solve one method simply by choosing another.

Alternative day method

The alternative day method is similar to the Eat-Stop-Eat and 5:2 method because it focuses on individual "on" and "off" days for fasting and eating. The difference for this method, in particular, is that you end up fasting at least 2 days a week and sometimes for 4 days. Some people follow very rigorous approaches to the alternate day method and fast every other day, consuming only 500 calories or less on fasting days. Some people, on the other hand, are much more flexible and tend to eat for two days, one day on an empty stomach, two days, one day on an empty stomach, etc. The alternative day method is even more flexible than getting up in that sense, since it allows the individual to choose how to alternate food and fasting, depending on what works best for the body and mind. The alternative day method is like a step up from the eat-stop-eat and 24-hour methods, especially if the individual alternates the fast of one day and the next day eating, etc. Surprisingly, this more intense style of fasting works particularly well for people who work in equally intense fitness regimes. People who consume more calories per day than 2000 (which is true for many bodybuilders and exercise enthusiasts) will have more to gain from the alternative day method since they only need to reduce their fasting diet to about 25 percent of standard caloric intake. Therefore, those fasting days can still provide solid nutritional support to fitness experts, helping them sculpt their bodies and maintain a new level of health.

Spontaneous omission method

The alternative day method and the Eat-Stop-Eat method are certainly flexible in their approaches to when the individual fasts and when he eats. However, none of the plans mentioned above are as flexible as the method of spontaneous omission.

Spontaneous jump method requires the individual to skip meals within each day, whenever you want (and when it is perceived that the body can handle it). Many people with sensitive digestive systems or practice regimens of more intense physical conditioning will start your experience with IF through the spontaneous jump method before moving on to something more intense. People who have very messy daily schedules or people who are around food a lot but forget to eat will benefit from this method, as it works well with chaotic schedules and unplanned energies. Despite this chaotic and disorganized potential, the method of spontaneous omission can also be more structured and organized, depending on what you do about it! For example, someone who wants more structure can choose which food each day they want to skip. Suppose you choose to skip breakfast every day. Therefore, your method of spontaneous omission will be structured around you, making sure to skip breakfast (that is, do not eat at least until 12:00 p.m.) every day. Whatever you need to do to make this method work, try it! This method is made for experimentation and adventure.

Crescendo method

The last method that is worth mentioning is the crescendo method, which is very suitable for the practice of women (since high-intensity fasts can be very harmful to their anatomy). This approach is made for internal awareness, soft introductions, and gradual additions, depending on what works and what doesn't. It is a very active type of trial and error method. Through the crescendo method, the individual begins to fast only 2 or 3 days a week, and on those days of fasting, it would not be a very intense fast. It would not even be so strict that the individual should not consume more than 500 calories, as with 5:2, Eat-Stop-Eat, and others. Instead, these "fast" days would be trial periods for methods such as 12:12, 14:10, 16:8, or 20:4. The remaining 4 or 5 days of the week would be open periods for eating. The professional is encouraged to maintain a healthy diet throughout the week. The Crescendo method works extremely well for female practitioners because it allows them to see how methods like 14:10 or 12:12 will affect their bodies without attaching them to the hook, line, and plumb line of the method. It allows them to see what each method does at the hormonal level, menstrual tendency, and mood swings. Therefore, the crescendo method encourages these people to be more in touch with their bodies before moving too fast towards something that can cause serious anatomical and hormonal damage. The Crescendo method will also work very well for overweight or diabetic professionals, as it will allow them to have these same "trial period" moments with everyone.

How to choose -- when choosing from the 10 different options listed above, there are several things to consider.

First, among these things will be the fact that you can always choose another method (or a more flexible one to start) in case something does not work as expected. In the end, you should also consider the following points when selecting your method: body type and capacity, lifestyle, daily trends, work routine, friends and family, and dietary options. For all these considerations, remember what you think is best and always remember to keep your goals in mind. If you ever have the feeling of sacrificing your sanity or physical health to achieve these goals, return to that problem-solving step, since you should never sacrifice those things to achieve any kind of goal. Keep an eye on the prize and remember to choose what is beautiful and see what works from there. Consider your body type and your skills.

Think about how your body looks and feels and how much you would like to change. Think about how you react to food and how it looks when you're hungry. Think of those things you see as "limits" and how comfortable you feel.

Are you a fitness enthusiast or a couch of potatoes?

Are you more hoarse or thinner?

Does your body retain fat or build muscles quickly?

Does it maintain the weight of water or not?

Do you exercise? Do you need much water when you do it?

Consider all these things about your body and more, then compare them with the methods listed above. Also, compare them to your general goals with intermittent fasting to make sure you choose a method that helps you update those goals as you conceive them. If you are looking to lose weight quickly, try a method that works with the "on" and "off" days between fasting and eating. If you are looking to build muscle, the lean gain method is probably the best option for you! If you are trying to stimulate your brain and heart, start with the crescendo method and see where it leads.

Consider your lifestyle.

 When do you get up normally, and how much do you sleep on an average night? How hungry are you normally when you wake up?

How fast is your metabolism, and when do you notice your peak?

How do you win at life?

Do you spend much time in the car, standing or in the office?

Are you constantly close to other people, or are you often alone?

When choosing the method of intermittent fasting, be sure to consider all these life points. You may not want to choose time with a method that does not allow you to eat when you usually need more energy. You may not want to choose a method that forces you to eat when you should be at work. Most of these methods have some degree of choice and flexibility, so when you find one that you like, remember that you don't have to put yourself in positions that go against your nature (or circadian rhythms) to achieve your goals. Be flexible, consider your goals, and respect the rules of your body!

Consider your daily trends.

Do you eat mainly during the day or after sunset? Do you work day or night? Do you usually stay home at night, during the day or at sunset? Do you have a lot of freedom and flexibility in your daily routines? Do you travel a lot for work? Do you spend much time on the move? Do you have trouble remembering to eat? Are you the type of person who practices regularly? Consider these problems in your life and more before choosing your method. Does it make sense to have days of low intake when you consume 500 calories or less? Or does it make more sense to have extended periods every day when you do not eat according to your habits or trends or whatever? Plan something that makes sense and respect your habits so that the transition to intermittent fasting is as simple and painless as possible. Consider your work routine. Are you going to work in the morning or the afternoon? Are you allowed to eat at work? Do you work in the food sector or the food services sector? Do you work on your feet all day or otherwise do something tiring? Do you have opportunities for intentional or accidental exercise at work, or are you sitting in the same position all day? All these elements of the work routine will be important to consider when deciding which path of intermittent fasting will be shortened. You won't want to participate in a method like 20:4 if you're at work every day for incredibly short shifts. The 20:4 method works best for someone who works very long and distracting days. You will not want to try a method like 12:12 if part of your window to eat involves being at work when you are not allowed to eat at work. Remember to take into account your work life, your routines, and restrictions when making this choice, as it will be much less difficult if you can see this larger image from the beginning and the planning stages.

Consider your friends, colleagues, and family.

How strong are your opinions? Are the lives of your friends health-oriented? Do they degrade you a lot or make fun of your choices? Or are they encouraging at all times? Are these people your support system, or are you the defender of your demons? Do you have the feeling that they want to see you succeed? At the most basic level, are they friendly to you and respectful of your choices? It may not seem so important, but the attitudes and supportive skills of your friends, colleagues, and family can mean the world when you make an important decision, such as starting an intermittent fast in your life. Sometimes people don't want to see us succeed. They block our successes with jealousy, pride, ignorance, or arrogance. When friends and family act in this way, it is best to choose a method that allows you to avoid talking about the IF. When friends and family are open and available, they should not influence your choice so much. It is only when things are weak that you will have to take them into consideration (and your time). Finally, consider your dietary choices. Do you eat a lot of processed foods? Or follow a diet based mainly on whole foods and vegetables? Do you count calories? Do you read nutritional data carefully? Are you looking for something specific like fat, fiber, or protein? Do you expect to change your diet completely or are you trying to keep things as they are? Are you willing to sacrifice elements of your diet to update your goals? All these questions help determine what type of method you will be prepared for. If you are looking to change your diet completely, a method of "days" and "days off" will work best for you. In this case, test 5:2, alternate days, consumption methods, feeding stops, and spontaneous emission. However, if you do not want to change your diet so much, a fasting method for periods within each day will be convenient. Try methods like 20:4, 16:8, 14:10, or 12:12 for this type of situation. Whenever you make your selection with these points in mind, you will surely achieve your goals of intermittent fasting. You allow yourself to choose the safest, smartest, and best option for your circumstances, and this is a fantastic tool to use in so many different applications. In this case, it is a tool that will help you stay healthy, stimulate your brain, heal your heart, and eliminate that excess weight like melted butter! As a reminder, your first option may not be the right one yet, but when you make the most courteous decision possible, you will definitely start from a good place and learn a lot about yourself independently. Make sure you have a final method (or two!) That is easy to change if the first seems to show no progress. Work smarter, not harder! Plan, research, and know yourself. These are the truest steps to success that I know. And as always, don't be afraid to consult your doctor or nutritionist once the decision is made. They can give you the last statement you need so you can start your new healthy lifestyle with intermittent fasting in no time!

Because women need intermittent fasting for women.

For those interested in losing weight, intermittent fasting may seem like an excellent option. However, many people would like to know if women should fast. Is intermittent fasting reliable for women? There have been a couple of studies exploring how intermittent fasting can help you lose weight in this fascinating new food trend. Intermittent fasting is also called alternative daily fasting, although there are some variations in this diet plan. The American Journal of Clinical Nutrition recently conducted a research study that included 16 overweight men and women in a 10-week program. On fasting days, people absorbed food up to 25% of their approximate energy needs. The rest of the time, they received dietary training; however, they were not given a particular criterion to meet during this period. What made this exploration fascinating is that many people need to lose even more weight than those who study the research before seeing the same settings. It was a fantastic discovery that encouraged a large number of people to try fasting. Intermittent fasting for women has some positive results. Women with a healthy diet and training strategy may have problems with persistent fat. However, fasting is a reasonable solution for this.

Intermittent fasting for women over 50 years old

Without a doubt, our bodies and our metabolic rate change when we reach menopause. One of the most important changes experienced by women over 50 is that they have a slower metabolic process and begin to gain weight. Fasting can be an unusual way to avoid this weight gain.

The studies try to show that this model fasting helps control hunger, and people who do not regularly experience the same aspirations of others. If you are over 50 years old and also try to slow down the metabolic process, recurring fasting can help you stop consuming too much daily. Your body also begins to establish some chronic conditions such as high cholesterol and hypertension when it reaches 50 years of age. Intermittent fasting has been shown to reduce cholesterol and blood stress, even without a fantastic offer of weight reduction. If you began to see your numbers improve every year in the doctor's office, you might have the opportunity to reduce them on an empty stomach, even without losing much weight. Recurring fasting may not be an exceptional idea for all single women. Anyone with a specific health condition or who often tends to be hypoglycemic should talk to a doctor. This new dietary pattern has special benefits for women who naturally store more fat in their bodies and may also have difficulty getting rid of these fat deposits.

Misconceptions about intermittent fasting (myths)

There is a lack of clinical thinking that justifies the 3 feeding methods per day, as current research studies reveal that fewer meals and even more fasting are adequate for human health and well-being. Intermittent fasting may be better if you eat 1-2 meals a day. Another myth is that serving breakfast is the most important meal of the day: in fact, there have been many erroneous cases involving the direct demand for a daily meal in the morning. The most normal claims are "the morning dish increases the metabolic procedure" and "the morning meal decreases the food intake during the day."

Effects of intermittent fasting on weight loss.

The uncontrolled desire to eat is caused by external forces. This occurs in times of war and shortage when food is limited. Food is easily served, but we choose not to eat it due to health and spiritual well-being or for other reasons. Fasting is as old as humanity, long before any other type of diet. Older people, like the Greeks, recognized that there was something naturally sensitive to routine fasting. Before the introduction of agriculture, people never ate 3 dishes a day plus intermediate snacks. When we find foods that can be separate days, we take them alone. From a development perspective, taking 3 meals a day is not a necessity to survive. Otherwise, we really shouldn't have endured it.

Fasting is inappropriate for service! Food manufacturers advise us to eat many dishes and take care of even one day. Fasting has no main period. It can be done from a few hours to several days or months. Recurring fasting is a food model in which one passes from one fast to another. Fasting has been done by millions and countless people for countless years. Numerous studies have revealed that it has enormous benefits for well-being.

What happens when we eat constantly?

Before combining the benefits of intermittent fasting, it is better to understand why eating 5-6 dishes a day or every two hours (exactly the opposite of fasting) can do even more harm than good. When we eat, we eat food energy. Fat causes less insulin effect; however, fat is almost never consumed alone. Insulin allows the body to start using nutrition quickly. Insulin transports glucose directly to the body's cells for use as energy. Healthy and balanced proteins do not necessarily increase blood sugar, but they can promote insulin. When the restriction is reached, the liver begins to convert sugar into fat. Subsequently, the fat disappears inside the liver (it also becomes fatty liver) or the first payments of fat in the body (regularly saved as persistent or persistent natural gastric fat). When we eat, in addition to a snack, during the day, we feed continuously, and insulin levels remain high. We could invest a large part of the day, keeping the power of food away.

What to expect from intermittent fasting

Intermittent fasting is a dietary pattern that alternates the duration of fasting and also manages to eat. It is a completely natural dietary technique divided into many types. Intermittent fasting approaches include fasting on alternate days, where an individual takes a typical diet on certain days of the week.

During fasting days, food is not avoided. However, calorie intake is reduced to 1/4 of the normal diet. The other type of fasting is that consumption is limited to a certain period within a day. The longest time a person can remain without food on intermittent fasting is 36 hours. For other conditions, intermittent fasting promotes essential health. It significantly reduces cravings for junk food and even sugar. This technique normalizes insulin in addition to the degree of sensitivity to leptin. Insulin resistance adds too many unstoppable health problems like diabetes mellitus, cancer, and heart infections. Intermittent fasting, therefore, will protect the body from such diseases. Intermittent fasting causes better mental well-being. The continuous breakdown of body fat causes the liver to create ketone bodies if it does not consume gains for some time. This type of fasting also improves the physical condition of the body and also promotes weight loss. Integrated fasting, in addition to training, increases the mobile aspects to optimize the breakdown of glycogen and fats. Exercising while hungry, for this reason, forces the body to dissolve stored fats to lose weight substantially. Also, the program aims to prevent cognitive impairment. The research was conducted in 2006 on mice, in which water puzzle tests were used to assess the cognitive characteristics of the mice on a regular diet plan, as well as those on recurring fasting. It was found that mice subjected to intermittent fasting experienced slower cognitive impairment, which is also used in humans. Recurring fasting will further increase muscle building, particularly in men. If the training is done during fasting, the body uses maintained body fat to maintain workouts. Finally, recurring fasting is a healthy practice. However, it can cause anxiety to people who fail to maintain it properly. Since only consistency will complete these positive results, commitment and resolution are needed to overcome dietary alterations.

Have you ever tried to reduce calories to lose weight? Did it work in the long term? Could you keep off the weight you lost? If you're reviewing this post, I guess it wasn't like that, and you are not the only one. According to the data of a British program, 1 of every 124 overweight women achieved results with this method. Take a quick look at what happened to the participants in the hit television series "The Biggest Loser." This program is an eternal example of why moving even more and eating much less works only temporarily. Why is it low in calories? Is there a bad diet prepared? A study of 14 participants in The Biggest Loser program showed some surprising results 6 years after the end of the show. The first results were excellent, and, as the research study revealed, they were short-lived.

Average weight before: 148 lbs / 328 lbs

Average weight after 30 weeks in the program: 90 kg.

Average weight after 6 years: 131 lbs / 131 kg

As you can see, the prospects lost much weight during the show; however, they have struggled to maintain weight loss for a long time.

Among the 14 who participated in the research study, they managed to maintain weight. This is more than a 95% deficit price! Then why? Review the detailed results below, revealing the incoming resting metabolic price (RMR).

Relaxation of metabolism

RMR reveals the amount of energy or calories the body burns to survive without movement. In some places, this is calculated in BMR or basic metabolic price. RMR is responsible for approximately 70% of all your metabolism, so the final results listed here are impressive.

• Average RMR before cooking: 2,607 kcal burned/day

• Average RMR after 30 weeks in the program: 1,996 kcal burned/day

• Average RMR 6 years after final weighing: 1,903 kcal burned / day. Despite the reality that participants returned about 70% of their first weight, their RMR did not return to pre-enrollment levels. It retained approximately 700 fewer calories per day! This indicates that to lose the same amount of weight in the second round, participants would need to eat 700 calories much less than the program. Because the initial diet contains 1200 to 1500 calories with 90 minutes of training 6 days a week. This would certainly be almost difficult. Why did RMR candidates continue to be so low even when they replaced the weight? The metabolic modification I have reviewed includes the BMR (basal metabolic rate) and also the RMR (resting metabolic price). Both explain how much energy (calories) your body uses to live without activity and represent approximately 70% of the entire metabolic process. This is not useful when the goal is permanent and lasting weight loss. Their results, once transformed, have remained stagnant and, in general, after the frustration that people offer and also all the accumulated weight, if they are lucky, their RMR/BMR will improve. Weight gain, making sure to return to what you lose with a steady yo-yo diet, can result in a lower metabolic rate that will fight to lose weight and may even be the heaviest you have ever been. Therefore, if eating incorrectly causes this, you will most likely wonder exactly how you cannot improve your intake in any way for a long period. Keep reading to see why.

Comparison of intermittent fasting for low-calorie dietary strategies

Reduced calories do not create hormonal changes in the fasting agent. They are the trick to lose weight and also their redemption. Other hormones that I have not indicated for reasons of simplicity are also stimulated during this start window to stop metabolic rate reductions related to low-calorie diet strategies. Low-calorie diet plans still include consumption, and even every time we eat, blood sugar levels will increase, activating insulin.

Summary

- Low-calorie diet programs can ruin the metabolic procedure making sustainable weight loss almost impossible.

- Maintainable weight loss depends largely on the regulation of hormonal agents.

- Fasting prepares the main hormonal agents for metabolic retention, muscle retention, and weight loss.

Why should you try intermittent fasting?

There are excellent offers of various diet programs to choose from. Some help you limit your carbohydrate intake and concentrate on large fats and healthy proteins. Some will limit your fat intake and also focus on healthy, balanced, and excellent carbohydrates. With all the alternatives in the industry, at least some of them are reliable selections to lose weight, so you may wonder why you should choose intermittent fasting. This portion will analyze the various benefits of periodic fasting and also how you will distinguish your health.

It changes the characteristics of cells, hormones, and genetics

Numerous things happen in your body when you don't consume for a while. Your body will begin to initiate procedures for cell repair work, as well as to modify some of its hormone agent grades, which will facilitate access to maintained body fat. Other adjustments that may occur in the body include insulin grades: insulin levels will reach a reasonable level, making it easier for the body to melt fat. Blood levels of human development hormone can increase significantly. This can help build muscle tissue and burn fat. The body will certainly begin important mobile repair procedures, such as removing all debris from cells. Some useful changes in innumerable genes will help you live longer and also protect you from disease.

Weight loss and body fat.

Many people take a quick flash to lose weight. In essence, fasting intermittently will help you, of course, to consume less food. You will certainly end up absorbing fewer calories, which will result in weight reduction.

Fasting improves hormonal function to help lose weight. Higher levels of the developmental hormone, in addition to reducing insulin, help the body break down fat, and use it for energy. That is why short-term fasting can increase the metabolic process by at least 3 percent. For one, it will improve your metabolism to make sure you burn many more calories by minimizing the amount you eat. According to a 2014 research study specialized in intermittent fasting, people could lose up to 8% of their body weight in less than 24 weeks. Help in Type 2 diabetes has proven to be substantial in recent decades. All that insulin minimizes resistance should help reduce your blood glucose levels and make sure that Type 2 diabetes stays away. Some show exactly how periodic fasting can help insulin resistance and also helps create a surprising reduction in blood glucose levels. In several research studies on intermittent fasting, blood sugar has been reduced by 3 to 6 percent, while insulin levels have been reduced by 20 to 30 percent.

A research study on diabetic rats also revealed that periodic fasting could protect the rat from kidney damage, which is a typical problem with many other extreme types of diabetes. This reveals that recurrent fasting could be an excellent option for anyone with a higher risk of developing Type 2 diabetes problems. There are some differences between the sexes. There is research that has revealed that blood sugar control can get worse for women after a periodic fast for a few weeks. We recommend that you talk to your doctor before starting any diet.

Speed up life

Although this cannot be considered an advantage in terms of well-being like the others, it is still essential to inform. Large groups find that intermittent fasting can make their lives less complex. They realize that they don't have to focus too much on the calories they consume, as long as they stay inside, and limit the hours they are allowed to eat. They can spend a few days a week without worrying about preparing a meal. In general, this diet plan can make life less complicated. When you can reduce some of the work you need to do during the day and emphasize something else, you can end up with less stress and anxiety in your life. We all understand how extreme stress can harm our well-being and our life. When you can reduce stress, it is much easier to be the healthiest variant of yourself. It can also be excellent for the heart. Heart disease is considered one of the most important diseases in the world. Periodic fasting can help with some of these threatening factors, such as lowering blood sugar levels, inflammatory markers, blood triglycerides, cholesterol, and hypertension. The most important problem is that many research studies on intermittent fasting have been performed on animals. We need to have even more studies that evaluate intermittent fasting and heart health in humans. It can also help with cancer. Many people have cancer every year. The uncontrolled advance of cells defines this horrible condition. It has been revealed that fasting has some exceptional benefits when it comes to its metabolic process, which can cause fewer threats to cells. Some human research studies reveal that fasting patients with cancer cells may reduce some of the secondary outcomes that include chemotherapy.

Useful for the mind

What is also considered fantastic for the body and mind? Intermittent fasting can help improve metabolic functions that help the mind stay healthy. This could include helping with insulin resistance, reducing blood sugar, reducing inflammation, and oxidative stress. Some rats have run in mazes that demonstrate how intermittent fasting can help stimulate the development of new afferent nerve cells, which improves mental function. Not eating can also help increase the degrees of neurotrophic appearance derived from the brain. When the brain lacks this, it can cause depression, along with other mental concerns.

Help for cell fixation

The cells of the body can begin to eliminate waste when we proceed in a rapid process recognized as autophagy, which implies that the cells break down and metabolize any healthy protein that cannot be used any longer. With a greater amount of autophagy, it could help protect the body from diseases such as Alzheimer's and even cancer.

It can prevent Alzheimer's Disease

Alzheimer's is among the most common neurodegenerative diseases. There is no cure for Alzheimer's, so the best step is to prevent it from happening as much as possible. A study in rats has shown that fasting intermittently can delay the onset of the disease of Alzheimer's or minimize its intensity. Reports have shown that a change in lifestyle that included some daily fasts or a minimum of regular temporary fasts helped improve the signs of Alzheimer's disease in 9 out of 10 patients. Research studies also show that things like fasting can help protect against other neurodegenerative diseases, such as the illness of Huntington's and Parkinson's. Intermittent fasting is a model, and research studies on how to make your body healthier are remarkably new. It will take some time to examine all the benefits of recurring fasting.

Intermittent fasting can help you live much longer

One of the most interesting attributes of periodic fasting is that it can help you live longer. In fact, there have been several research studies on rats looking at this.

Intermittent fasting can help prolong its lifespan, comparable to what happens when you have a constant calorie limitation. In some research studies, the impacts have been surprising. In one of them, when mice did not eat every two days, they end up living 83 percent more than mice that did not fast. It was really difficult to reveal an increase in life expectancy because periodic fasting has not yet been analyzed in people with enough time to identify it, it is still a prominent concept for those seeking to stop aging. Since there are recognized benefits to the metabolic price with this diet, it is not uncommon for people to think that intermittent fasting can certainly help them live a much longer and even healthier life.

As you can see, there are many advantages to choosing a repetitive fasting diet. Let's take a look at some of them. However, many research studies have been conducted on the results of this diet plan and why you can benefit from it. If you are looking to improve brain health, live much longer, lose weight, or gain even more energy, periodic fasting can improve your life.

Three factors essential to take into account

1. Set goals

You must have a clear vision of what you want to achieve. Vague goals like "I want to get fit," "healthy and balanced" or "lose a few extra pounds" will not be enough when things get tough. Make a clear variable to do this or stop the possibilities. These points are worth considering;

What do you want to do that you can't do now?

➢ 30 days

➢ 12 months

How do you want to look?

➢ 30 days

➢ 12 months

How would you like to feel inside?

➢ 30 days

➢ 12 months

After solving this, it is also advisable to ask yourself why you want these things and what will undoubtedly be different if you achieve these goals. This will help you understand what is critical for you. Many times our goals originate in the consequences for outdoor living; however, in the end, they must interact with you. Review your information and establish a:

➢ 30-day goal

➢ 90-day goal

➢ 12-month goal

If you need help setting goals, be sure to join my personal Facebook community.

2. Organization

Analyze your agenda! I often see that people choose a window in their day to eat only to discover that they do not have time to consume during this period. It is not a great start! Analyze where you may have difficulties without food. If you have a monotonous dining room, it is probably not practical to configure your home window on an empty stomach during the slowest part of the day. If dining with the house is a routine, leave it in the consumption window. Be sensitive when choosing your energy window. Make this procedure as simple as possible on your own.

3. Support

It is necessary to surround yourself only with beneficial people who undertake the same specific trip. It will be difficult, and sometimes you will want to quit. Having others to support it is necessary to succeed, and it could be the difference between the two. You give up or follow the battle! Feel free to join my FREE online support system here.

Element 1: diet and nutrition.

As you will probably understand, nutrition plays an important role in any health and fitness trip. The important thing is that we often know what to eat! We know that vegetables are useful for you, meat has protein, and you probably know that processed foods are generally bad. I will not offer you the usual thing to avoid bread, pasta, blah, blah, spiel, which you have heard hundreds of times. We will cover two essential electrolytes essential for weight loss that is normally lacking in people, as well as the amount of fat, protein, and carbohydrates that you should take to get the best results. Remember that, in the beginning, focus on getting used to the window of your house. You will get immediate results when you are used to transferring the 16:8 lifestyle with much more sophisticated suggestions for additional results.

Fats, carbohydrates, and proteins.

As mentioned earlier, the goal of the game is to burn glycogen stores by forcing the body to use fat. Over time, the goal is to get used to our bodies. Burn fat as the main source of gas to stay thin throughout the year. The best way to do this is to limit carbohydrates and also improve fat intake. It is worth it. Healthy proteins should be kept at a moderate level since most of them can be converted directly into sugar, and the body also stores them as glycogen. Here are some common macro examples.

I want to take this opportunity to emphasize that it is not necessary to be Keto or follow a ketogenic diet to obtain results with IF. Always be sure to consult your doctor before transforming your diet.

Fat: 50%

Protein: 30%

Carbohydrates : 20%

Fat : 60 %

Protein: 30 %

Carbohydrates: 10 %.

Fat: 65%

Protein: 25%

Protein guidelines

When trying to lose weight a normal mistake is to drink a lot of protein. As discussed earlier, excess protein can be converted into sugar and maintained as glycogen. Due to the difference in atomic composition, sugar cannot be transformed into protein. Use the formulas provided to calculate healthy protein needs based on your goal.

Weight loss = 0.36 g-- 0.7 g per kilo of body weight OBJECTIVE.

Instance: Mandy estimates 198 pounds but has a nominal weight of 174 pounds.

0.36 x 174 = 62.64.

0.70 x 174 = 121.8.

The ideal daily intake of Mandy protein varies from 62 g to 122 g.

Mandy would make sure she had at least 62 g of protein per day.

Your muscles are safe. However, they do not require more than 122 g per day to prevent healthy proteins from converting to glucose.

Volume = 1.5 g-- 2 g per kilo of body weight OBJECTIVE.

Example: John estimates 165 pounds; however, he has a nominal weight of 200 pounds.

1.5 x 165 = 247.

5.2 x 165 = 330.

John's perfect daily intake of healthy proteins is more likely to be between 247 and 330 g. Certainly, John is more likely to need supplements, since the amount of food needed to reach this amount of protein can be unbearable for consumption. As the volume increases, it is typical for the body fat section to improve; however, when the target weight is acquired, a reduction phase is certainly performed.

Carbohydrate Guidelines

Carbohydrate calculation can be difficult, as it differs from one person to another.

Here are some standards that can be met. Keto = 30 g or less each day.

These should come mainly from green leaves.

This method is a concept extracted from the ketogenic dietary strategy.

Destroyer of the highlands = 100 g or less every day.

These should come mainly from resistant starches and also from green leaves.

This concept is valuable if you have reached a plateau. Beginner = Eliminates refined sugars.

Instead of focusing on macros, the beginner's emphasis should be to eliminate refined sugars and complement immune starches.

Immune starches.

They are immune to the digestion of food and function as a soluble fiber.

They help reduce blood sugar levels and insulin resistance. These are many much better options than traditional carbohydrate options.

Examples are: sweet potatoes and sweet potatoes instead of white potatoes.

Oatmeal instead of cereals.

Cooked and cooled rice instead of hot rice.

Green bananas instead of other fruits.

Fat guidelines

Some people still find it difficult to understand that fat consumption is not transferred instantly to "gain weight."

As Nina Teicholz exposes in her book "The Big Fat Surprise," the low-fat movement is full of false information and dubious clinical assistance. I advise you to read her book. If you want to burn fat as a fuel to lose weight forever, you will have to accept eating much more fat than you think healthy. I do not say that you should go to the keto, but the constant consumption of saturated fats (yes, you have read it correctly) will help your body to burn fat as fuel. AVOID trans and hydrogenated fatty oils. Partially hydrogenated oils include trans fats. The trans fats triggers a series of various health problems, including an increase in "bad" cholesterol.

Fruit patterns

There are many contradictory details about fruit that should have a special reference in this publication. The basic fact is that fruit is rich in sugar.

At the molecular level, your cells do not divide foods like fruits and chocolate into a "healthy and balanced" classification, as well as "unhealthy and balanced."

Sugar is sugar, period. Any other type of sugar, fructose, dextrose, and many other words that end in "bone" are transformed into glucose and used as necessary. The fruit should be eaten seasonally and also in extremely small quantities if you are trying to lose weight. Our bodies are connected to use the fruit as a representative volume for the colder months when food will certainly be limited. Our bodies do not realize that we live in a culture where we have access to food throughout the year. A fruit being sent to your body must pass conservation status as the winter season approaches. That's how fruit suggests you use when trying to lose weight.

I have tried fruit smoothies.

Drink fruit immediately after training with a protein shake. Never consume fruits without a protein source. Healthy fruit smoothies are sugar bombs. The amount of sugar cancels any antioxidant effect the drink may have.

Fruit is an excellent means of improving insulin so that muscle cells can absorb the protein shake.

Breakfast guidelines

A more controversial issue that is entitled to a special recommendation is breakfast. You've probably heard that breakfast is one of the essential meals of the day. However, this is completely wrong. YOU HAVE NO BREAKFAST IN THE MORNING. The word breakfast only means breaking the fast. From now on, please think of the morning meal as the first dish of the day, regardless of when you eat it. I have a morning meal from 1:00 pm to 2:00 pm. Traditionally, people have found it much easier in 16:8 to open the window to start eating later in the day. The most notable idea I can give you when it comes to what your real starter food is. Make sure it is rich in protein and healthy fats but low in carbohydrates. The element for this is that everything you initially consume will identify the claims that your body will disperse during the day. A carbohydrate-rich breakfast will prepare the body to look for sources of sugar, which will provide unpleasant cravings for sugar, low energy, and a cloudy brain. A morning meal rich in protein and healthy fats will prepare the body to look for fat for gas and keep it full for longer. It has also been revealed that starting the day with this type of morning meal helps fight stress and anxiety by promoting higher levels of serotonin. The fruit well trembles with ecological alternatives to the leaves. Get rid of cereals for foods like eggs and avocados. Feel free to pour some grass-fed meat directly into the mixture. Prevent immune starches in this meal.

Summary

Use the formula indicated in the protein standards to calculate your daily protein needs accurately. Immune starches are better for blood sugar levels and also announce the level of insulin sensitivity. Preparing foods with hydrogenated fats is healthier than using hydrogenated oils such as oil. It is hydrogenated fat if it remains solid at normal room temperature. Pet supplies for grain feeding are wild and even undesirable. Eating fruit without a protein resource increases blood sugar and insulin. Breakfast involves breaking the fast. Not eating in the morning will not make you fat. Your first course should be a high healthy protein and fat.

Electrolytes

These bad habits add numerous characteristics to our bodies, from contraction to sending messages between the mind and the body's organs. To offer you the best possible start without disturbing you, we will most likely talk about 2 crucial electrolytes that can start contributing to your diet today.

Potassium

When we have muscle pain, we are often informed that we have no water and magnesium. Currently, this is true. However, an additional reason for muscle stiffness could be a lack of potassium. This is because we are asking for much more potassium per day than magnesium.

Some signs of low potassium content may include:

➢ Muscle tension.

➢ Swollen ankles.

➢ Sugar cravings (yes, a reduction in potassium can cause sugar cravings).

Some sources of potassium.

➢ Beet tops.

➢ Avocado.

➢ Spinach.

➢ Lima Beans.

➢ Pope.

➢ Brussels sprouts.

Try to include some of these in your dietary strategy much more regularly to increase your potassium. There are no potatoes, as they have a high carbohydrate content. These are still better in percentage.

Magnesium

As you probably already understand, low magnesium content can trigger muscle pain. It is fascinating to note that an excellent supply of magnesium from food is lost throughout the process of digestion of food. Salted rock and magnesium creams are an excellent technique to ensure that muscle mass becomes sufficient. Some signs of magnesium reduction may include:

➢ Muscle discomfort.

➢ Difficulty sleeping.

➢ Stress and also anxiety.

Some sources of magnesium:

➢ Spinach.

➢ Almonds.

➢ Quinoa.

➢ Sesame seeds.

The most common mistakes and how to solve them

Intermittent fasting is an excellent process that can lead to exemplary health effects. However, any process can only work efficiently if its execution is correct, and no mistakes are made in the execution. This chapter will explain some of the most common mistakes made by women during intermittent fasting. This chapter will focus on the basic mistakes we make at random, but that can dramatically damage our weight loss and health goals. Pay attention to macronutrients. This is one of the most important things to remember. People who suffer from obesity want to get rid of this malice. They are ready to change anything for this. They dream of a slim figure as their ultimate goal, and this is where they run the risk of making some of the fatal mistakes. Intermittent fasting or any form of diet or caloric restriction would impose some restrictions. Intermittent fasting does not limit the amount of food you can eat or its type. However, this does not mean that you can eat a lot. In most cases, you will only have between 7 and 8 hours to eat what you want. While it may seem like a long time, you will find that the time for the final meal of the day is approaching long before the previous meal has been digested. Losing that meal may mean you will have to go without food until the next meal. Therefore, the amount of food you can eat is limited. Other calorie limiting routines place an explicit limit on the amount and type of food you can have. These things have a profound impact on your health. You may experience weight loss, but that does not mean you are recovering. Your body can only recover when you receive all macros and micronutrients in the correct amount. It would help if you also had vitamins and minerals. Achieving this while consuming limited calories can be difficult. If you do not pay proper attention here, you will end up with nutritional deficiencies. You can get a thin frame, but you will have more problems than when you started. The best way to combat this problem is a properly balanced diet. Intermittent fasting gives you the right opportunity to do so since it does not impose restrictions on the amount and types of food you may have.

The best way to overcome this trick with qualifications is to have a very balanced meal. Your meals should be high in fat, moderate in protein, and low in carbohydrates. Before I begin to question the credibility of the suggestion, I would like to clarify some misconceptions: fat is not bad, but there is a popular misconception that eating fat is bad. Fat is the cornerstone of life. It has some important roles in our life. Our bodies cannot function without fat. Fat, in general, is not bad.

The trans or low-quality fats that we get in processed foods are bad. Fat itself is a form of compact energy. Our body does not classify food as fat, protein, or cholesterol. Everything you eat is transformed and divided into calories. This means that fat would also be converted to glucose, and this would happen with carbohydrates. The advantage of eating fat is that you can eat more calories in a single meal than carbohydrates. Fat is very compact and has almost twice the calories per gram of carbohydrates. So, if you get 8 calories per gram of carbohydrates, you will get 16 calories of fats. Protein is also heavier and has more calories than carbohydrates. This means that if you follow a diet high in fat and low in carbohydrates, you can get more calories. It also means that even if you eat fewer meals a day, you will not have a shortage of energy. Fat should be consumed in large quantities. It is necessary to select high-quality fats. The same goes for proteins. You can get protein from animals and cereals, and it would help you build muscle and stay fit. The biggest advantage of having a diet high in protein, and low in carbohydrates, is that it doesn't make you feel hungry very often. The fat and protein content in your meals will help you easily switch from one meal to another without addressing the need for snacks. Diets rich in fats and proteins also contain many minerals and vitamins. However, most minerals, vitamins, and fiber must be obtained from carbohydrates. You should consume many green leafy vegetables, salads and whole foods. The green leaves are bulky and do not weigh much. They don't add too many calories to your system, but they provide most of the vitamins, minerals, phytonutrients, antioxidants, and trace elements your body needs. You can have all the green leafy vegetables you want without worrying about calories. They are rich in fiber and, therefore, keep the digestive system healthy and also improve immunity. This is a part that should never undermine your search for a slim figure. If you ignore your health, your weight will return faster than you can lose it. It will also have a very negative impact on your health. It would help if you always remembered that you need to be healthy to lose weight and that it is not the other way around. People who lose weight drastically without a solid foundation are called sick and unhealthy. It would be best if you never forgot the macronutrients in your food, as they would become the pillars of your health.

Don't be greedy in festive windows

Food has its temptation. It seems the most attractive in the world when it has been private for a long time. But it is important not to be greedy in those moments and lose control. It is very important to leave the windows fasting properly. The biggest mistake people make is that they eat a lot after breaking the fast. This can cause several problems, and poor digestion is one of them. On an empty stomach, the intestine stays away from food for prolonged periods and, therefore, can dry up a bit. Filling it with heavy foods can cause problems. The best way to start the day is to start with liquid foods and then switch to semi-solid and solid food. You should also consider the amount of food you eat. Our brain takes much longer to understand the signs of leptin that indicate we are full. When your brain tells you that you are full, you would have eaten too much. The best way out is to eat slowly, as this would give the brain time to assess satiety levels. You can also stop eating when you think you are 80% full.

All in all, you will have eaten enough. If you want to try this, you can wait a while after feeling 80% full, and you will discover that you are no longer hungry. It occurs when fat cells can communicate properly with the brain that it is no longer necessary to eat.

Do not try to speed up the process.

Slow and steady wins the race. This is an adage that we have all heard, but most of us do not believe it. We want fast results, and for this, we are ready to jump. However, this is not how the body works. Your body travels very slowly. You need time to adapt to any positive or negative change, and the same would happen even in the case of intermittent fasting. If you want to succeed with the process, you must make sure you complete all the steps for a while. You have to give your body time to adapt. There are habits of decades that should change, and sometimes it can be difficult for your body. If you want your body to react favorably to change, you should not rush the process. Fasting in men and women is completely different. Men have a very resistant system and are not affected by a slightly extended rapid program. However, this is not the case with women. If you try to shake the system a little harder, this can negatively affect your health. Your hormonal system can change, and normalization can take a long time. A woman's body reacts very differently to the signs of stress and, therefore, caution and patience are essential. Start with the simplest process and give your body time to adapt to small breaks. Once you are accustomed to a certain amount of fasting, try to stretch it a bit slowly. Do not do anything very fast. Always go step by step, and you will reach your goal easily and without unnecessary difficulties.

Perseverance is the key

Impatience is a big problem in people struggling with weight. There is no fault since they are subject to strong pressure. Most people trying to lose weight have already faced disappointments with other weight loss measures and, therefore, want to see the results quickly to believe it. They are not ready to wait long for the results. This is a point where problems can occur. Intermittent fasting is a wonderful process, but it does not work by magic. Try to correct problems that may have reached their current state of development in the past. The results will take time to arrive. You will have to work with patience and not lose hope when the results arrive. If you stop smoking in the middle, you cannot know if you are progressing or not. It is not a process that works overnight. A leap of faith will be required, and you will devote your time and energy.

Don't frame unrealistic expectations

We all like to dream big, and that is a good thing. However, we must also remain based in reality. This will help to accept the facts and save many disappointments. Many times we are so caught up in imaginary expectations that we don't recognize the gifts we receive. If your goal is weight loss, think about the amount of time you are ready to devote, the distances you can travel, and the medical conditions you face. Without considering all these facts, expecting a complete makeover would be absurd. If you have met these expectations, you will not even be able to enjoy the weight loss you are observing. Your expectations would overshadow the results. It is important to stay realistic.

Properly manage your fasting time

It is not unusual for some people to mishandle their time. Many of us do it in our daily lives. However, bad time management can cause serious difficulties. It can make your weight loss journey difficult and painful. You can't keep thinking about food while you fast. This will create problems for you, and your gut would also be confused. The best way to manage your fasting time is to keep busy. The last part of the fasting window should always be programmed to remain locked correctly. The more inactive you are, the more likely you are to think only of food. Performing intense physical activity is one of the best ways to postpone hunger. Hunger in the current era is a highly psychological phenomenon. Our bodies have ample reserves of energy to function without food for months. It is our mind that always attracts us to food. You have to stop it for a few hours. Walking, running, laughing, talking with friends, starting serious discussions are some of the ways we can stop hunger and not be affected. These are some of the most common mistakes we make that can ruin the results we get. Intermittent fasting is a very simple and easy way to lose weight. It doesn't take much time and effort. You only have to decide once and take it in your life. Even if you are following some other measure of weight loss, intermittent fasting can adapt to your lifestyle.

Differences between young and old

At the most basic level, it should be said that there are detailed body differences between young women and older women. Many of these bodily differences are manifested by the external physical effects of aging, but many also occur within, far from what our eyes can see. As women age, enter, and leave menopause and mature fully, their bodies change, reflecting different nutritional needs for the next 30 years. During menopause, in particular, some foods help with impulses, hot flashes, and more, but the period of intense transition is more a door to a completely altered future (mental, physical, nutritional, and more). Women of this age experience a slower metabolism (with great frustration) and a decrease in hormone production. For weight and mood, therefore, menopause and maturation are equal disasters. Your body will become completely "out of control" compared to how it used to work. You are likely to gain weight despite the dietary choices you make, and you may feel that there is no relief in sight. Don't be fooled, however! Things may have changed for you, but they won't be stagnant changes. Basically, women in menopause and beyond need to absorb less energy in general from their food, but they need more protein to cope with the effects of aging. It will be necessary to increase vitamins B12 and D, calcium, and zinc, while iron becomes less important for the aging of the female body. Vitamins C, E, A, and beta-carotene should also be increased to fight cancer, infections, diseases, and more. As women get older and mature, more things will change; mainly, it is no longer possible to give up these important supplements. In older and more mature women, the body's ability to recognize hunger and thirst is silenced, and dehydration represents a serious threat. Fewer calories are needed even for the older and more mature woman, but she still needs to eat as many nutrients (if not more!) than the young woman. It seems that a younger woman can eat (relatively) what she wants and not worry about taking vitamins or supplements, but it is undeniable that the older woman will need this nutritional help to ensure longevity. Health needs become more pressing for women at this age, since their bodies are less flexible and resistant to problems that may arise.

How IF affects women at this age and how to handle it

As health, diet, reproducibility, and nutritional needs change for mature and menopausal women, their relationships with intermittent fasting can be very different from those of young women. For example, while young women should pay attention to how intermittent fasting can affect their fertility levels, older women can freely practice intermittent fasting without these concerns. Therefore, older women can apply intermittent fasting weight loss techniques to their own lives without worrying about the negative side effect that may arise in the future. However, for menopausal women, the situation is slightly different from that of fully mature women. Women who go through menopause are dealing with daily hormonal fluctuations that cause hot flashes, insomnia, anxiety, irregular periods, and more. At the beginning of this process, intermittent fasting will not necessarily help and may even make your situation more stressful. For women in this situation who are actively going through menopause, they should remember that their body is extremely sensitive to changes at this time. If you find that intermittent fasting helps and that short periods of fasting are effective, you should also make sure to increase the intensity of fasting as gradually as possible so that your body can adapt without creating horrible hormonal repercussions for you and everyone else. For a fully mature woman, intermittent fasting will not make you feel moody, irregular in your period, or otherwise because those hormones will no longer affect you, or at least, not a great deal. Their dietary choices are released more than the effects they have had on hormonal health over the years. Therefore, if you are trying to lose weight, have better energy, a physiological shake to regain health, or whatever you have, try IF without worries and see what happens. For these types of women, intermittent fasting is set to provide hope through reduced depression, a lower chance of cancer (or recurrence), promised weight loss, and more.

Tips and tricks for women over 50

As we have seen in the previous topics, intermittent fasting is not easy. We need all the support and everything that can facilitate your trip. Here are some tricks that will facilitate your trip.

i. Decide your fasting window.

Intermittent fasting is not a strict time-based diet. This means that you can choose the number of hours to fast and when to fast day or night. The periods of fasting and feeding do not have to be the same every day.

ii. Make sure you get enough sleep.

When you get enough sleep, you become healthier, and your overall well-being is guaranteed. When we sleep, the body performs certain functions that help burn calories and improve metabolic rate.

iii. Eat healthily.

Avoid eating what you want after a fast. Healthy meals should be the center of attention. They will help you get the necessary nutrients, such as vitamins, that will give you more energy during the fasting period.

iv.   Drink more water.

One of the best decisions you can make during a fast is to drink water. It will keep the body hydrated and drinking water before meals can significantly reduce appetite.

v.   Start with something small.

If you have never tried it before, there is no way to start fasting and spend 48 hours without eating. To start, you can start eating at 20:00, for example, and you will have nothing left until 8:00 the next day. It will be easier because the dream is integrated into your window to eat.

vi.   Avoid stress.

Flickering can be difficult to do if you are stressed. This is because stress can trigger excessive food indulgence for some people. It is also easier to feed on garbage when stressed to feel better. That is why in intermittent fasting, it is recommended to avoid, if not control, stress levels. Be disciplined. Remember that fasting means withdrawing food for a while. When fasting, be true to yourself and avoid eating before the appointed time. It will ensure that you lose maximum weight and benefit from intermittent fasting in healthy terms.

vii.   Keep drinks flavored.
The most flavored drink says they are low in sugar, but in reality, they are not. Flavored drinks contain artificial sweeteners, which will negatively affect health. They will also increase your appetite, which will cause you to overeat, and this will cause you to gain weight instead of losing.

viii.   Find something to do when you fast.

It is said that an inactive mind is the devil's workshop. When you fast intermittently and are not busy, you will think about food, and this will prevent you from fasting before the set time. You can run errands, listen to music, or even take a walk in the park.

ix.   You can train while fasting, but it is not mandatory.

Mild exercises can also be done at home. When you train, you will develop muscle strength, and body fat will burn faster.

The best exercises to lose weight after 50 years of age

Physical activity is the last part of the triad of weight loss, but it is no less important. Exercise pumps blood, releases endorphins during and after workouts, and can help you burn extra calories. The number of calories burned will depend on the type of exercise, duration, and intensity. However, it is generally a small amount and does not approach the number of calories burned by the basal metabolic rate. The average Joe will not have the time or resources to devote significant attention to calorie consumption.

Instead, exercise helps in other ways. In the case of intermittent fasting, it can help regulate energy levels and deplete available glycogen stores, forcing the body to burn fat if it is not already. Do you remember those old-school exercise videos with everyone who talked about "burning"? Exercise will rarely burn fat directly. Fat only burns after glycogen stores are depleted (which takes some time). Most amateur athletes never reach that level of performance.

Sometimes we think that burning some calories (for example, 3,500) is equivalent to burning 1 kg of fat. More specifically, it is burning 3,500 calories, resulting in the loss of a pound of fat, more or less. Many people believe that exercising on an empty stomach is harmful to you. One way this could be true is to cause a significant drop in blood sugar levels. Here, diabetics have to be very careful. The best time to train would be only a few hours after starting a fast when the energy of food is still in the body. An exercise of any kind naturally reduces blood sugar levels. If someone cannot regulate their blood sugar levels efficiently (diabetes), they run the risk of having a severe episode of hypoglycemia. Otherwise, the body can detect that blood sugar levels are decreasing and give an adequate response to metabolize glycogen. People who have difficulty training during fasting may choose to "cheat" when they have a small meal before training. Protein shakes are known for this, as they tend to be rich in carbohydrates and proteins. Mixing whey protein with water can vary between 120 and 400 calories, depending on the amount of powder used. Mixing it with milk will significantly increase the caloric content. But you usually don't need protein shakes to exercise.

If you are already used to the fat-burning phase of a low carb diet, it will be easier for you to train regularly, even on an empty stomach. Trying to do a complete workout during the first week of Keto will be difficult. Trying to train in the middle of a fast is also difficult because you will suffer the symptoms of low blood sugar. People with diabetes should take precautions against it. Since a person with diabetes should regularly monitor blood sugar levels, he should schedule a blood meter test just before deciding to exercise. If your blood sugar level is too low, you should not exercise. At a minimum, they should eat something so that these levels return to a healthy interval for physical activity. As with fasting, training should end if symptoms of dizziness, vomiting, or loss of consciousness occur.

The types of exercises you decide to perform will depend on your fitness goals. A good general recommendation for people who want to be healthier is resistance training at least twice a week, along with the recommended 150 minutes of moderate to intense aerobic activity. These 150 minutes can be further increased to 300 minutes to receive even more benefits. These include reducing the risk of cardiovascular disease, reducing the risk of cancer, and increasing the weight loss potential of physical activity alone. If a full 300-minute exercise is sustainable per week while fasting will depend on the person's fitness level and the appearance of their fasting routines, for example, someone who is doing the "5:2" method can only decide No Train on your fast days, others who skip breakfast every day (and fast overnight) may decide to finish training at the end of the fasting period. Breaking the fast with a small meal and then training later is a good option. The exercise becomes a bit more complicated with longer fasts (1-3 days or more). The considerations remain the same, and the risk of hypoglycemia episodes increases.

Benefits of exercise.

While exercising on an empty stomach can be expected to present a challenge, there are many benefits. First, exercise without food in the system means that the calories consumed directly affect glycogen stores. In the short term, this means that you will lose weight quickly from the water stored in glycogen and accelerate fat burning. In addition to burning glycogen, you can expect cellular processes to burn at least some fat. They are called AMP kinases and are responsible for accelerating the metabolism of fat in the muscles during workouts. They burn the fat when the body detects that there is enough energy to avoid calories from sugar. The true essence of what happens during quick exercise can get complicated quickly, but your body secretes all kinds of things. Muscles that are exposed to excessive oxidative stress from exercise during fasting become resistant to that stress over time, avoiding the rhythm of the aging process. The brain and muscle tissues go into a rejuvenation process similar to autophagy that keeps things running smoothly. These effects are mainly stimulated during short and intense workouts, such as HIIT workouts and resistance training.

Small amounts of human growth hormone (HGH) are released even if you train when glucose stores are low. In turn, this stimulates the secretion of androgens such as testosterone that nourishes the libido and increases lean muscle mass.

Aerobic exercise

Everything that rises and moves is considered aerobic. In particular, it is about increasing your heart rate for prolonged periods. It comes from the word that means "with oxygen," which makes you breathe faster than normal, providing your body with enough oxygen to flow into the blood. Walking, jogging, jumping rope, biking, climbing stairs, and countless sports qualify for aerobic exercise. Current guidelines on physical activity in the United States recommend at least 150 minutes of this type of exercise per week. One of the easiest things you can do is walk. Walking is virtually free in most cases and can be a pleasant change of pace. You can bring your dog or friend to accompany you. Fast aerobic exercise will use glycogen primarily as fuel, depending on how fast it is. If you train immediately after the last meal, you can get an energy boost. Believe it or not, people who exercise in their fasting period report higher energy levels than a non-fast workout. This has to do mainly with HGH body secretion, among other things, to compensate for the lack of readily available energy. But these energy levels are generally reserved for people who are accustomed to fasting. If you try to train during the first weeks of testing, expect great resistance from your body. It is advisable to take things slowly and gradually increase the intensity or duration of fasting workouts. Meanwhile, you can train on days without fasting as usual.

Anaerobic exercise

The opposite of aerobic exercise is the anaerobic type. This covers various forms of resistance training, including bodyweight exercises, strength conditioning, and weightlifting. High-intensity workouts such as HIIT and sprint training are also covered. Anaerobic exercise and resistance training, in general, are good for building muscle and strengthening bones. The nervous system also benefits from the mind-body connection used with resistance training. Resistance effectively teaches muscles how to interact with brain signals. Both anaerobic and aerobic exercise should be used together to obtain maximum weight loss results. The main difference between the two is that, under anaerobic conditions, the oxygen that enters the body through the lungs is not enough energy to maintain training. Instead, muscles need to break down sugars (glycogen) to get the energy they need. This decomposition provides weight loss by reducing the amount of glycogen available anytime. Broken glycogen stores lead to the accumulation of lactic acid, which is the main reason why muscles feel sore after intense training. The breakdown of muscles also causes a repair mechanism not only to repair torn muscle fibers but also to remove dead components from cells. It would help if you recognized it immediately as autophagy. You will experience an increase in metabolism that lasts hours after training, fasting, or not. The basic rule for exercising during fasting is not to push things. If dizziness, migraine, vomiting, etc. occur at any time while training, it is not a challenge to continue, but a signal that you should stop. This is especially true if you train in a warm climate since the temperature will cool your body during overtime.

Hydration is important since dehydration is an important cause of heatstroke. If you plan to lift heavy weights for anaerobic exercise, be sure to exercise lighter than normal on fasting days. Lifting heavy objects with insufficient glycogen stores is a good way to pass out in front of everyone in the gym.

Recipes

Greek breakfast covers

This recipe is as satisfying as the fast-food breakfast sandwich. However, this compress has much less fat and fewer calories. It is a quick breakfast to prepare in advance and warm up early in the morning or when you get to work.

Ingredients:

- 1 teaspoon olive oil.
- 1/2 cup fresh spinach leaves
- one tablespoon fresh basil
- four egg whites, whipped.
- 1/2 teaspoon salt
- 1/4 teaspoon freshly ground black pepper
- 1/4 cup low-fat crumbled feta cheese.
- 2 whole wheat tortillas (8 inches).

Instructions

In a pan, heat the olive oil over medium heat. Add spinach and basil to the pan and fry for about 2 minutes, or only until the spinach dries. Add the egg whites to the pan, season with salt and pepper and cook, gently stirring, for another 2 minutes, or until the whites are firm. Remove from heat and sprinkle with feta cheese. Heat the tortillas in the microwave for 20-30 seconds, or only until they are soft and hot. Divide the eggs between the tortillas and finish the burrito style. Makes 2 servings.

Avocado and fennel salad with balsamic vinaigrette

This salad contains a wonderful mix of tasty citrus, soft avocado, and aniseed fennel. Mixed with a quick and direct balsamic vinaigrette, it is the best light lunch or dinner for hot days. It contains 250 calories.

Ingredients:

- One tablespoon of light olive oil.
- One tablespoon balsamic vinegar
- 1/4 teaspoon salt
- 1/2 cup fennel, sliced
- 1/2 avocado diced
- 1/2 cup mandarins, drained.
- 1 cup sliced romaine lettuce
- 1/4 teaspoon freshly ground black pepper

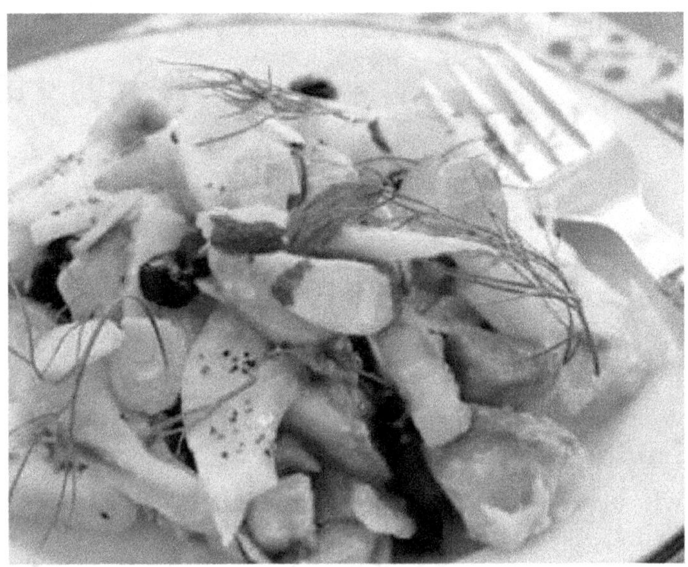

Instructions

In a medium bowl, add olive oil, balsamic vinegar, salt, and pepper, and mix until well combined and slightly thick. This is your balsamic vinaigrette. Include fennel, avocado, oranges, and lettuce; Stir until the vegetables are well covered with a dressing. Divide between 2 salad plates and serve cold. Makes 2 servings.

Zucchini Omelet

Preparation time: 4 minutes

Cooking time: 3 hours and 30 minutes.

Servings: 6

Ingredients:

1½ cups chopped red onion

1 tablespoon olive oil

2 cloves garlic minced

2 teaspoons chopped fresh basil

6 beaten eggs

A pinch of sea salt and black pepper

8 cups sliced zucchini

6 ounces fresh tomatoes, peeled.

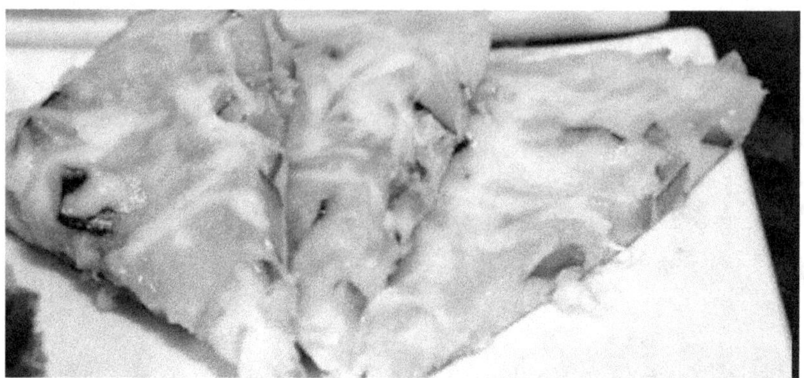

Instructions:

In a bowl, mix all ingredients except oil and basil. Grease the slow cooker with the oil, distribute the tortilla mixture in the bowl, cover, and simmer for 3 hours and 30 minutes. Divide the tortilla between the dishes, sprinkle the basil, and serve for breakfast.

Chile Tortilla

Preparation time: 5 minutes

Cooking time: 3 hours and 30 minutes

Servings: 4

Ingredients:

- 2 cloves of garlic minced
- 1 tablespoon of olive oil
- 1 chili pepper
- 1 small yellow onion, minced
- 1 teaspoon of chili powder
- 2 tablespoons of Salsa de tomato
- ½ teaspoon of sweet paprika
- A pinch of salt and black pepper
- 1 tablespoon of parsley,
- 4 chopped eggs, beaten

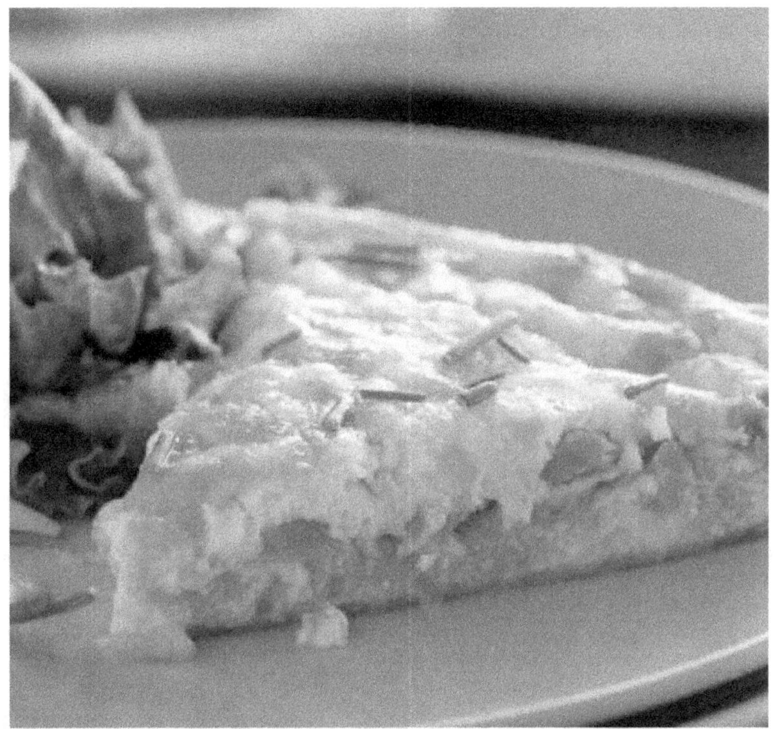

Instructions:

In a bowl, mix all ingredients except oil and parsley and beat them well. Grease the slow cooker with the oil, add the egg mixture, cover and simmer for 3 hours and 30 minutes. Divide the tortilla between the dishes, sprinkle the parsley, and serve for breakfast.

Penne With Vegetables

Even on fasting days, you can enjoy a light meal of pasta. It is full of vitamin C, spinach, and tomato and offers a lot of flavor and satisfaction. (200 calories per serving)

Ingredients:

- 1 teaspoon salt, divided.
- 3/4 cup raw penne.
- 1 tablespoon olive oil
- 1 tablespoon chopped garlic
- 1 teaspoon chopped fresh oregano.
- 1 cup sliced fresh mushrooms

- 10 cherry tomatoes, cut in half.
- 1 cup fresh spinach leaves
- 1/2 teaspoon freshly ground black pepper
- 1 tablespoon grated Parmesan cheese.

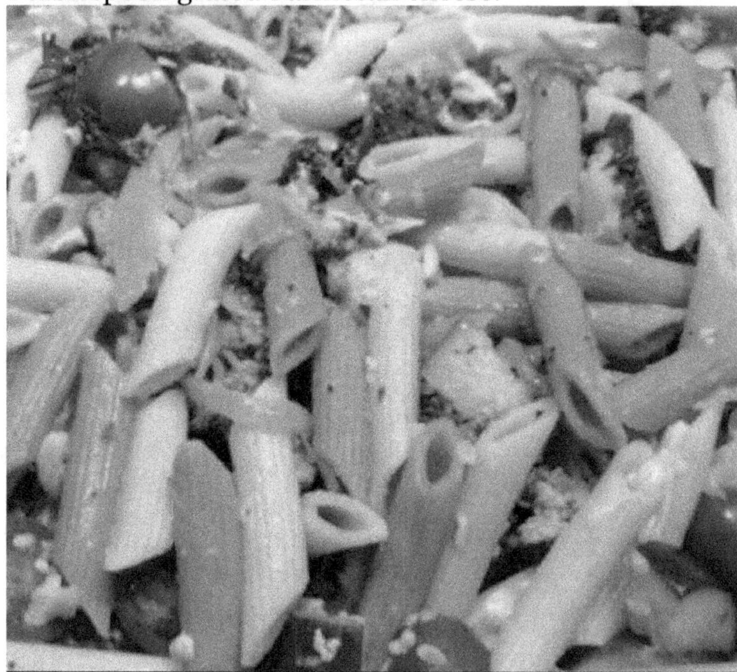

Instructions

In a large skillet, pour 1 liter of water until it boils. Include 1/2 teaspoon of salt and penne and cook according to package directions or up to approximately 9 minutes. Drain but do not wash the penne, keeping approximately 1/4 cup of pasta water. Meanwhile, in a large skillet, heat the olive oil over medium-high heat. Include garlic, oregano and mushrooms and fry them for 4-5 minutes or until the mushrooms are golden brown. Add the tomatoes and spinach, season with the remaining 1/2 teaspoon of salt and black pepper and brown for 3-4 minutes or until the spinach melts. Add the drained pasta tubes to the pan, along with 2-3 tablespoons of pasta water. Cook, constantly stirring, for 2 or 3 minutes, or until the pasta shines and the water has not cooked. Divide the pasta into 2 shallow bowls and sprinkle with Parmesan cheese. Serve hot or at room temperature. Makes 2 servings.

Breakfast with basil and cherry tomatoes

Preparation time: 4 minutes

Cooking time: 4 hours

Servings: 4

Ingredients:

- 1 tablespoon olive oil
- 2 yellow onions, chopped
- 2 pounds cherry tomatoes, cut in half
- 3 tablespoons tomato sauce
- 2 cloves garlic minced
- One pinch of sea salt and black pepper
- 1 bunch of chopped basil

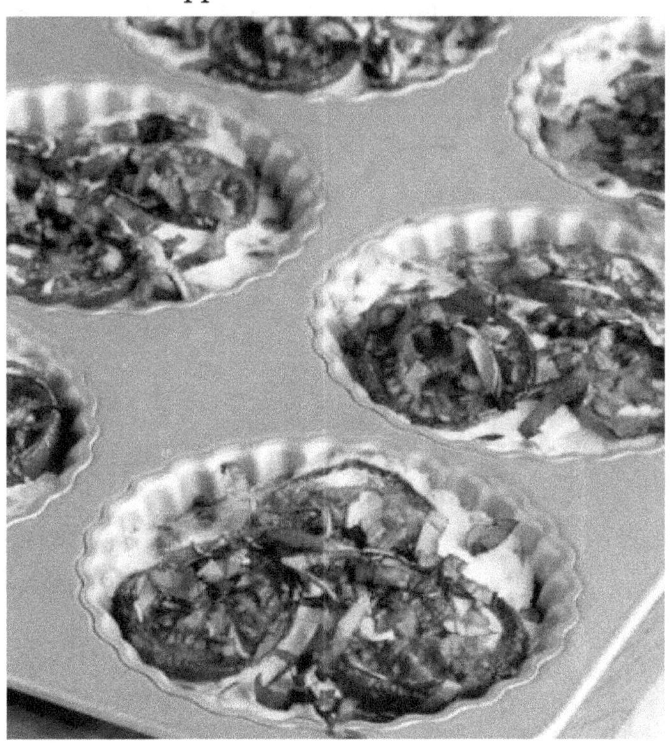

Instructions:

Grease the slow cooker with oil, add all the ingredients, cover and cook over high heat for 4 hours. Stir the mixture, divide it into bowls, and serve for breakfast.

Carrot salad

Preparation time: 5 minutes

Cooking time: 4 hours

Servings: 4

Ingredients:

- 2 tablespoons of olive oil
- 2 pounds of carrots, peeled and cut in half
- 3 cloves of garlic, chopped
- 2 yellow onions, chopped
- ½ cup broth Vegetables
- 1/3 cup crushed tomatoes
- A pinch of salt and black pepper

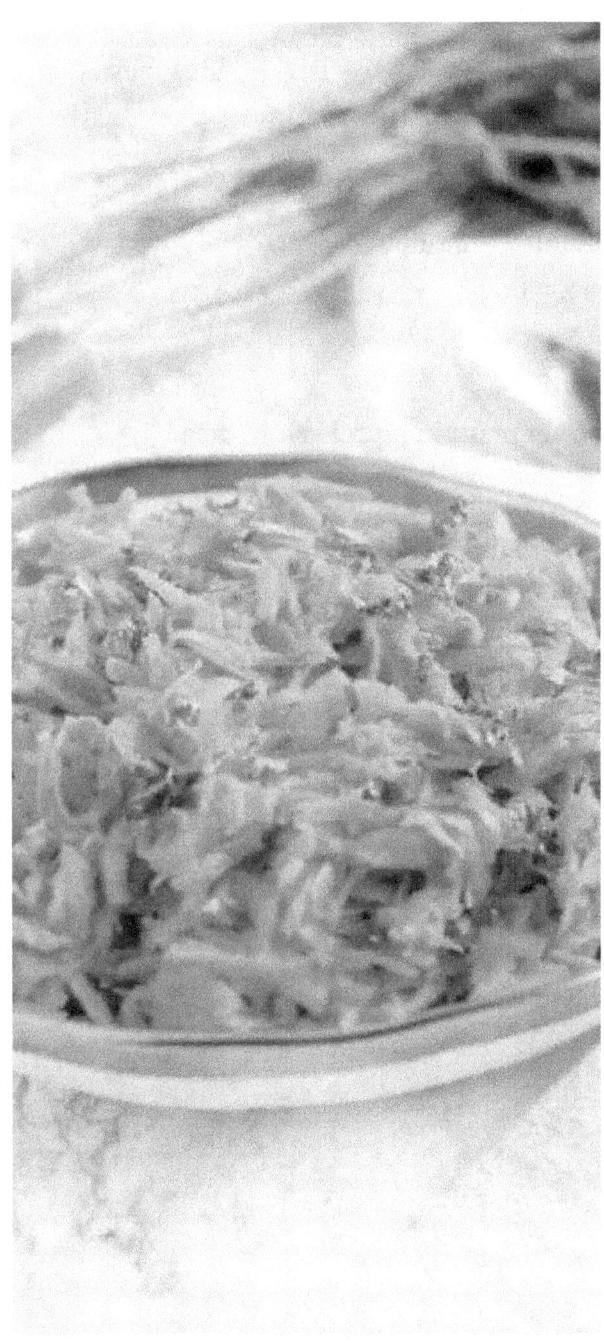

Instructions:

In the slow cooker, combine all the ingredients, cover and cook over high heat for 4 hours. Divide into bowls and serve for breakfast.

Sweet Pumpkin Mix

Preparation time: 5 minutes

Cooking time: 7 hours

Servings: 6

Ingredients:

- 6 kilos of pumpkin, peeled and diced
- 1 cup apple cider
- 1 teaspoon ground cinnamon
- 1 teaspoon grated fresh ginger
- ½ cup grated maple syrup
- A pinch of chopped nutmeg

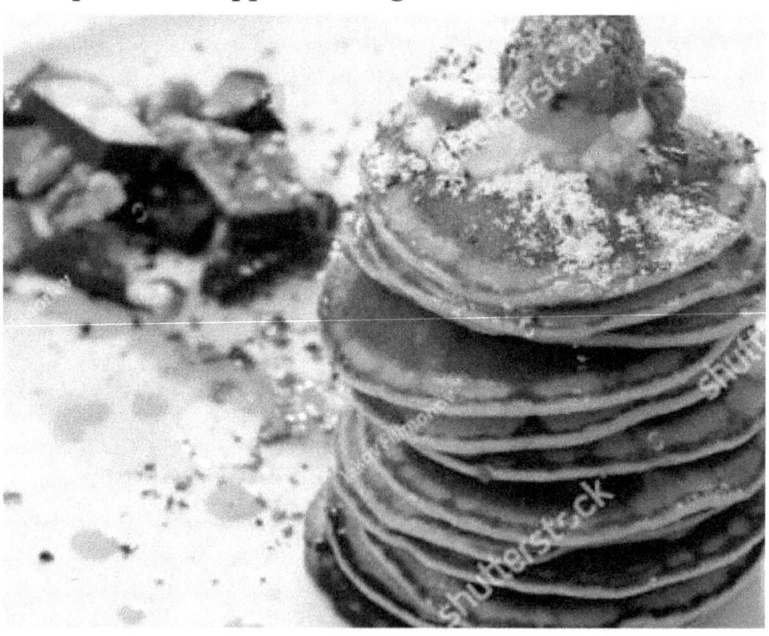

Instructions:

In the slow cooker, mix all ingredients, cover and simmer for 7 hours. Divide into bowls and serve for breakfast.

Balsamic Onion Jam

Preparation time: 5 minutes

Cooking time: 4 hours and 15 minutes

Servings: 6

Ingredients:

- 2 tablespoons olive oil
- 4 pounds yellow onion, sliced
- ½ teaspoon baking soda
- 5 cloves garlic, minced
- ½ cup water
- ¼ cup balsamic vinegar
- 1 teaspoon dried thyme
- A pinch of salt and black pepper
- 1 teaspoon red pepper flakes
- 2 tablespoons coconut sugar

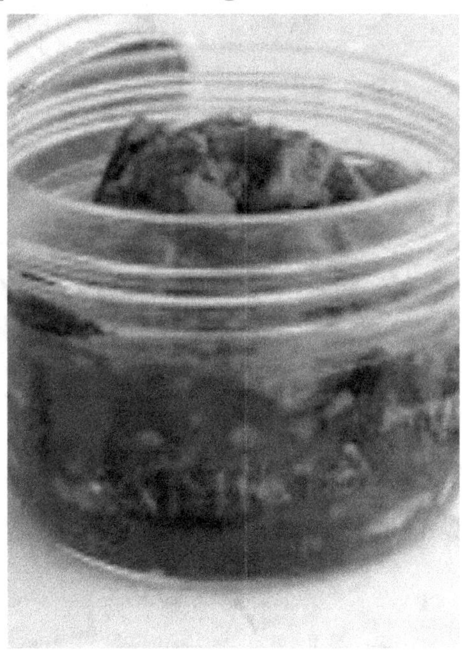

Instructions:

Heat a pan with the oil over medium heat, add the onions and baking soda, stir fry for 15 minutes and transfer to a slow cooker. Add the rest of the ingredients, beat, cover, and simmer for 4 hours. Mix the jam, divide it into jars, and serve at breakfast or at any time of the day.

Zucchini and Garlic Mix

Preparation time: 5 minutes

Cooking time: 6 hours

Servings: 6

Ingredients:

- 4 cups zucchini, sliced
- 2 tablespoons olive oil
- 1 teaspoon Italian seasoning
- A pinch of salt and black pepper
- 1 teaspoon garlic powder

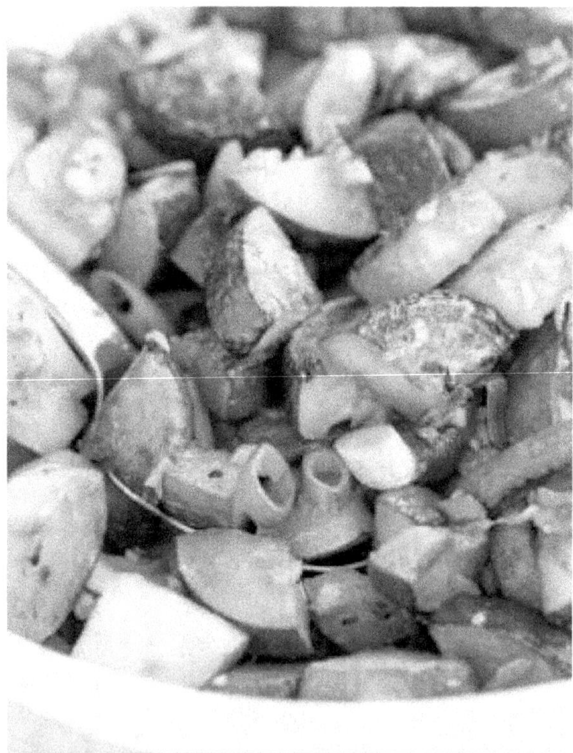

Instructions:

In your slow cooker, mix all ingredients, cover and simmer for 6 hours. Divide into bowls and serve for breakfast.

Spinach and Swiss Cheese Omelette

It is not necessary to reserve tortillas for breakfast or breakfast. An omelet can be an excellent option for dinner on the busiest nights and is also a rewarding lunch on weekends. (150 calories per serving)

Ingredients:

- 1 teaspoon olive oil
- 6 large egg whites, whipped
- 1 cup fresh spinach leaves
- 1/2 teaspoon salt
- 1/4 teaspoon freshly ground black pepper
- 2 slices (1 ounce) of low-fat Swiss cheese.

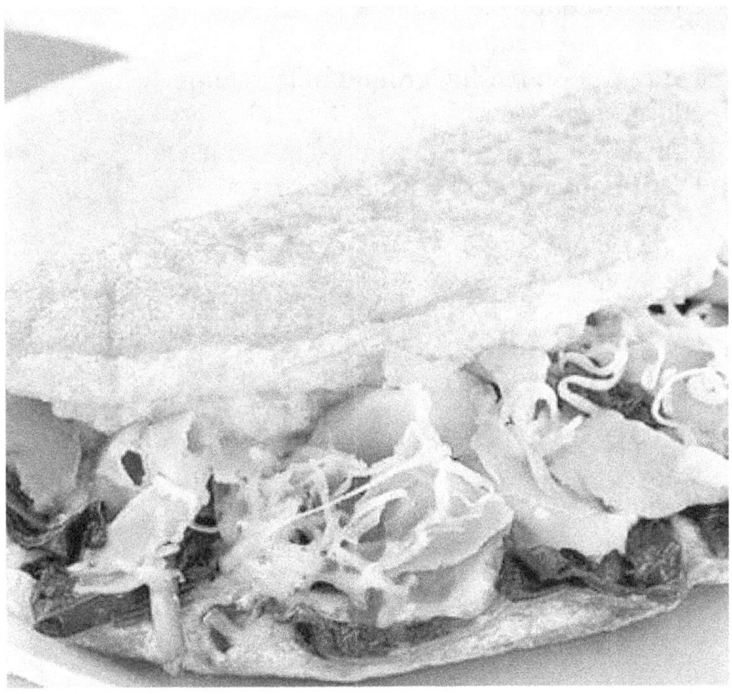

Instructions:

In a pan, heat the olive oil over medium-high heat. Add spinach, salt and pepper and fry them for 3 minutes, stirring frequently. Use a spatula to distribute the spinach evenly in the bottom of the pan and pour the egg whites over, tilting the pan to cover the spinach completely. Cook for 3-4 minutes, periodically pulling the edges of the eggs towards the center while tilting the pan to allow the raw egg to cook the edges of the pan. When the center of the eggs is almost dry (but not completely), use a spatula to rotate the eggs. Place the slices of Swiss cheese in the middle of the tortilla and turn the other half forward to form a crescent. Cook for 1 minute or until cheese melts and heats. To serve, cut the tortilla in half and serve hot. Makes 2 servings.

Parmesan egg toast with tomato

This breakfast is quick to prepare and delicious to eat. You can replace grape tomatoes if you have them on hand. They provide a healthy dose of vitamin C (150 calories per serving).

Ingredients:

- 1 teaspoon of olive oil
- 1/2 teaspoon sliced garlic (about 1 clove)
- cherry tomatoes, in quarters.
- 1/2 teaspoon salt
- 1/4 teaspoon freshly ground black pepper
- 2 large eggs
- 2 pieces of low-calorie whole-grain toast.
- 1 tablespoon grated Parmesan cheese.

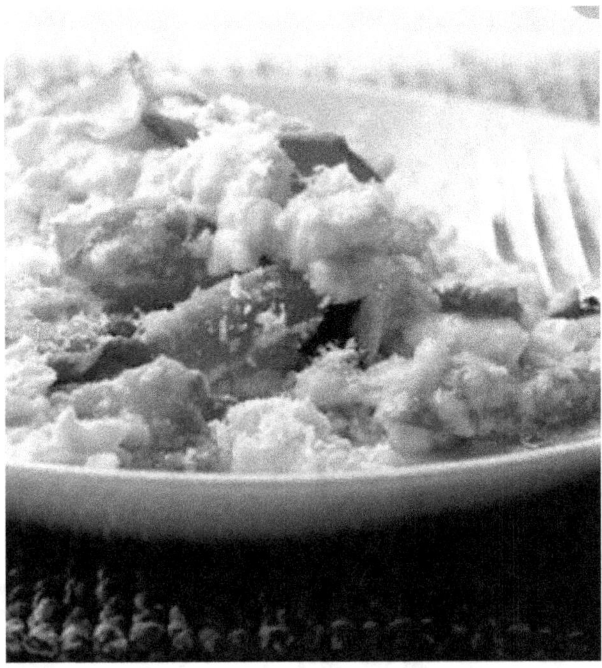

Instructions:

In a pan, heat the olive oil over medium heat. Add the garlic and tomatoes to the pan and fry them for 2 minutes, stirring occasionally. Season with salt and pepper, then switch to a hot plate. In the same pan, fry the eggs for 2 minutes. Turn and cook at the desired temperature (30 seconds easier, 1 minute for more than half, 2 minutes better). Put 1 egg on each piece of toast, with half the tomatoes, and sprinkle with half the parmesan. Makes 2 servings.

Lamb sirloin with turmeric

Preparation time: 15 minutes

Cooking time: 16 minutes

Servings: 4

Ingredients:

- 13 ounces of lamb
- 1 tablespoon of turmeric powder
- ½ teaspoon of chili flakes
- 3 tablespoons of olive oil
- 1 tablespoon of balsamic vinegar

- 1 teaspoon of salt
- ½ teaspoon of peppercorns
- ¾ cup of water

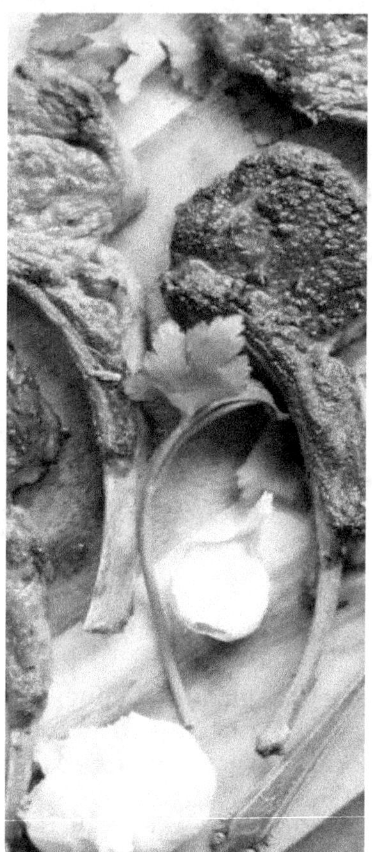

Instructions:

In a shallow bowl, mix the turmeric powder, chili flakes, olive oil, balsamic vinegar, salt, and peppercorns. Generously brush the lamb with the mixture. Then preheat the grill to 380F. Place the lamb grill on the grill and cook for 8 minutes on each side. The cooked lamb grill should have a slightly crunchy crust.

Sausage Casserole

Preparation time: 10 minutes

Cooking time: 35 minutes

Servings: 6

Ingredients:

2 jalapeno peppers, cut

5 ounces of cheddar cheese, grated

9 ounces of sausages, chopped

1 tablespoon of olive oil

½ cup spinach, chopped

½ cup cream

½ teaspoon of salt

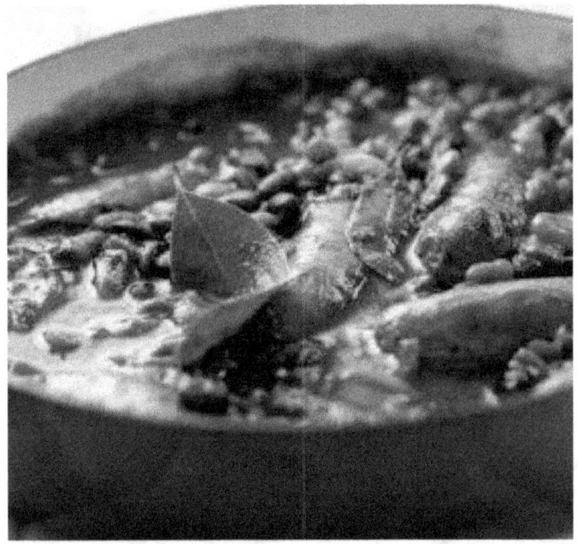

Instructions:

Brush the pan with olive oil. Then put the chopped sausages in the cake pan in a layer. Add chopped spinach and sprinkle with salt. Then add the sliced jalapeño. Then prepare the layer of grated cheddar cheese. Pour the thick cream over the cheese. Preheat oven to 355F. Transfer the pan to the oven and cook for 35 minutes. Use the kitchen torch to blacken the cheese.

Baked salmon fillets with tomatoes and mushrooms.

Salmon is an excellent source of healthy fats, especially omega-3 fats. Baked with a mixture of spicy tomatoes and moderate mushrooms, it is as delicious as it is healthy (200 calories per serving).

Ingredients:

- 2 (4 ounces) of salmon fillets with skin.
- 2 teaspoons of olive oil, divided.
- 1/2 teaspoon salt
- 1/4 teaspoon freshly ground black pepper.
- 1/2 teaspoon sliced fresh dill.
- 1/2 cup diced fresh tomatoes
- 1/2 cup sliced fresh mushrooms

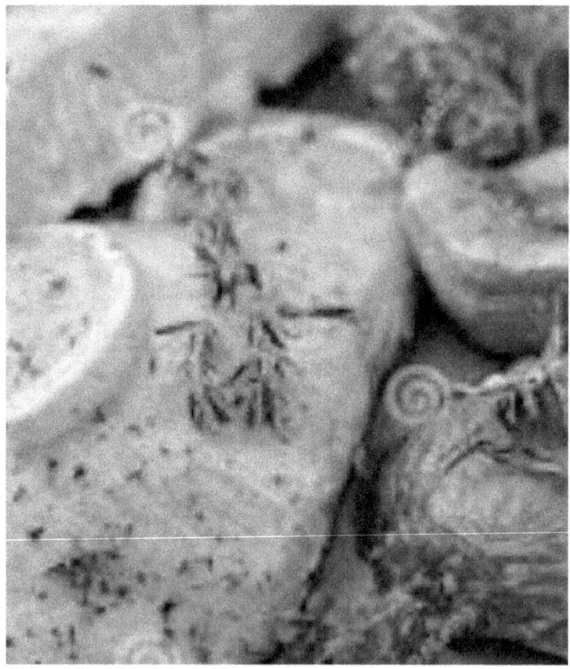

Instructions:

Preheat oven to 375 degrees F and cover a baking sheet with foil. Using your fingers or a pastry brush, cover both sides of the fillets with ½ teaspoon of olive oil each. Put the salmon with the skin facing down. Sprinkle evenly with salt and pepper. In a small bowl, combine the remaining 1 teaspoon of olive oil, dill, tomato, and mushrooms; mix well to integrate it. Place the mixture on the fillets. Fold the sides and ends of the leaf to seal the fish, place the pan on the central grill and cook for about 20 minutes or until the salmon crumbles quickly. Makes 2 servings.

Sweet Protein Potatoes

This dish is very simple and fast. However, it loads almost 10 grams of protein per serving, making it an ideal meal for a quick day to keep it full and help it stay stimulated and concentrated (200 calories per serving).

Ingredients:

- 2 medium sweet potatoes.
- 1/2 teaspoon salt
- 1/4 teaspoon freshly ground black pepper.
- 6 ounces of natural Greek yogurt.
- 1/3 cup dried cranberries

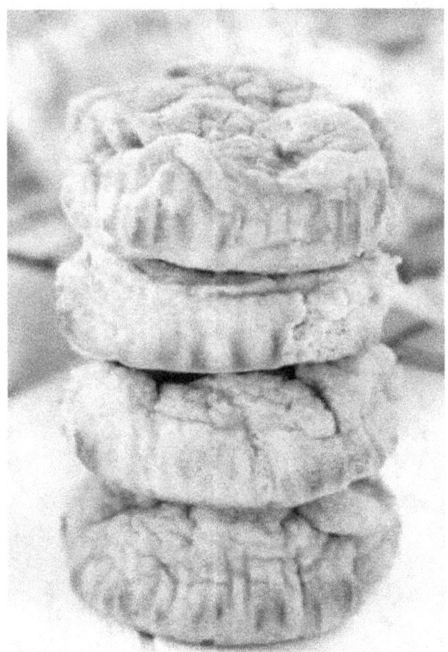

Instructions:

Preheat oven to 400° F and pierce sweet potatoes several times with a fork. Place them on a baking sheet and cook for 40 to 45 minutes, or until they can be easily pierced with a fork. Cut the potatoes in half and place the meat in a medium bowl, keeping the shells intact. Add salt, pepper, yogurt, and blueberries to the bowl and mix well with a fork. Replace the mixture in the potato peels and serve hot. Makes 2 servings.

Miso soup with Chinese cabbage and prawns

If you like Asian flavors, you will love this quick and easy soup. It cooks in a couple of minutes, making it an excellent recipe for your busiest nights. It overheats well, so it is also an excellent option for a business lunch. (150 calories per serving)

Ingredients:

- 2 cups of water.
- 8 large raw prawns (34-40 beads), peeled and cut in half.
- 1 cup of bok choy cut into slices.
- 1/4 cup white miso paste.
- 1 cup of diced corporate tofu.
- 2 green onions, sliced.

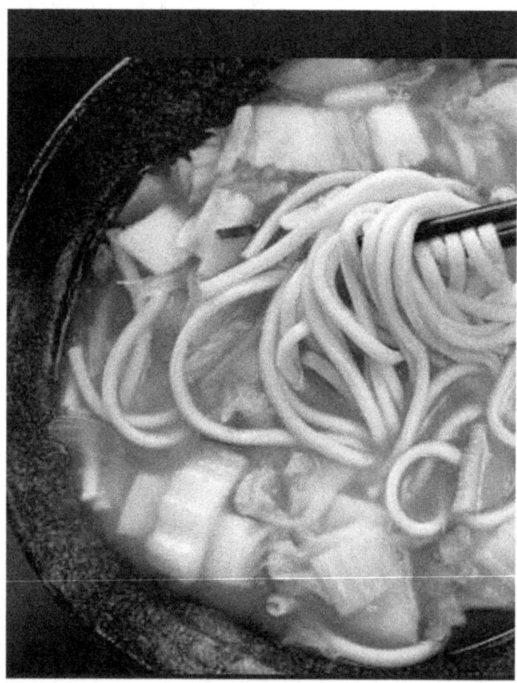

Instructions:

In a medium saucepan, boil water over high heat. Add the prawns and boil for 1 minute. Reduce heat and add Chinese cabbage. Boil for 2 minutes, then add miso and tofu. Boil for 1 more minute. To serve, divide 2 bowls of soup and sprinkle with green onion. Makes 2 servings.

Cajun pig sliders

Preparation time: 10 minutes.

Cooking time: 45 minutes.

Servings: 4

Ingredients:

- 4 slices of low-carb bread
- 14 ounces of pork tenderloin
- 2 tablespoons of Cajun seasoning
- 1 tablespoon of olive oil
- 1/3 cup of water
- 1 teaspoon of tomato sauce

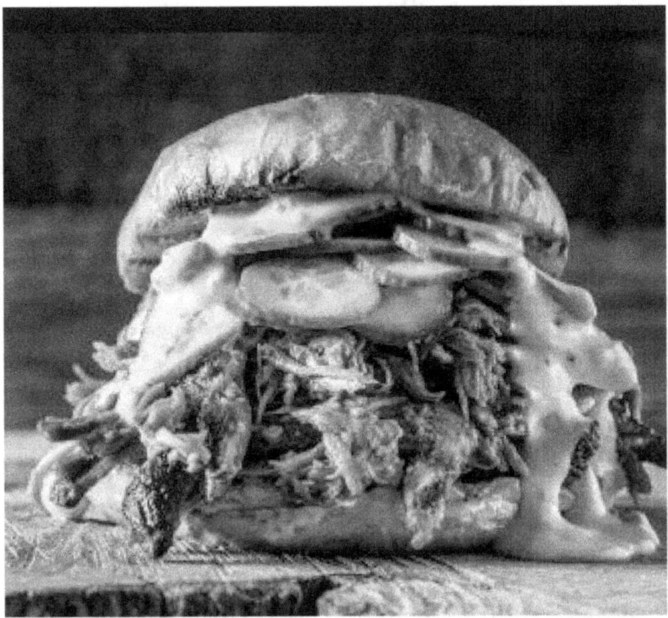

Instructions:

Rub the spicy pork loin Cajun and put it in the pan. Add olive oil and roast over high heat for 5 minutes on each side. Then, transfer the meat to the saucepan, add the tomato sauce and the water. Stir gently and close the lid. Boil the meat for 35 minutes. Cut the cooked pork loin. Place the pork on the slices of bread and transfer them to the serving plates.

Grilled halibut with garlic spinach

Halibut is a deliciously moist fish that is rich in heart-healthy omega-3 fats. If you replace frozen halibut, be sure to thaw it completely and give it an extremely dry pat before cooking. (200 calories per serving)

Ingredients:

- 2 halibut fillets (4 ounces) 1 inch thick.
- 1/2 lemon (about 1 teaspoon of juice).
- 1 teaspoon salt, divided.
- 1/4 teaspoon freshly ground black pepper.
- 1/2 teaspoon cayenne pepper
- 1 teaspoon olive oil.
- 2 cloves of garlic.
- 1/2 cup sliced red onion
- 2 cups fresh spinach leaves.

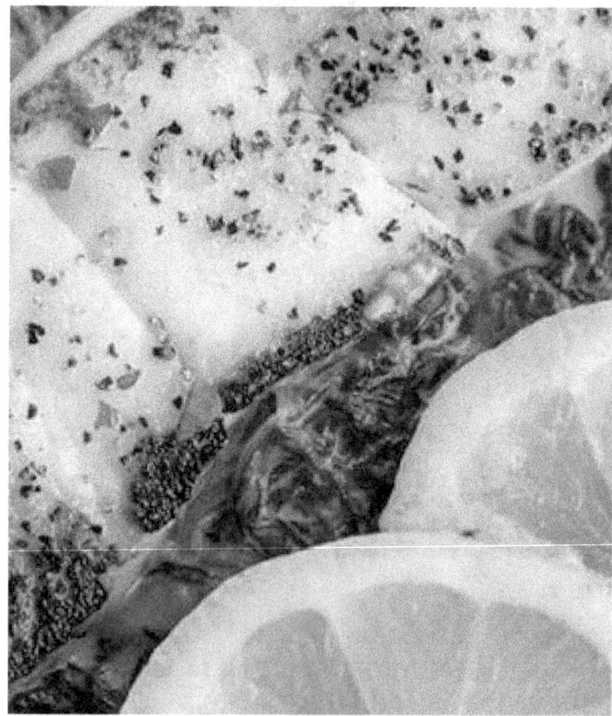

Instructions:

Preheat the grill and place a 4 to 5 inch grill under the heat source. Line a tray with a baking sheet. Squeeze half of the lemon over the fish fillets, then season each side with ½ teaspoon of pepper and salt. Put the fish in the pan and roast for 7 to 8 minutes. Turn the fish over and roast for another 6-7 minutes or until it wobbles. Meanwhile, heat the olive oil in a pan over medium heat. Add the garlic and onion and fry for 2 minutes. Include spinach and half a teaspoon of salt and brown for another 2 minutes. Turn off heat and cover to keep warm. To serve, divide the spinach between two plates and cover each serving with a fish fillet. Serve hot. Makes 2 servings.

Beef tenderloin stuffed with sticky sauce

Preparation time: 15 minutes

Cooking time: 6 minutes

Servings: 4

Ingredients:

- 1 tablespoon of erythritol
- 1 tablespoon of lemon juice
- 4 tablespoons water
- 1 tablespoon butter
- ½ teaspoon ketchup
- ¼ teaspoon dried rosemary
- 9 oz beef fillet
- 3 oz grated celery root
- 3 oz sliced bacon
- 1 tablespoon chopped walnuts
- ¾ teaspoon minced garlic
- 2 teaspoons of butter
- 1 tablespoon of olive oil
- 1 teaspoon of salt
- ½ cup of water

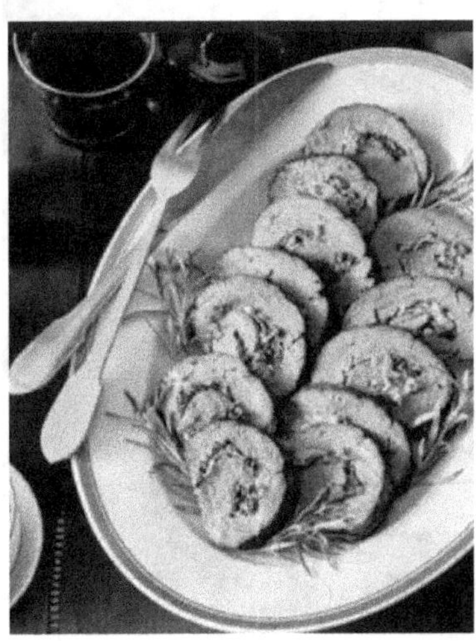

Instructions:

Cut the beef fillet in layers and spread with dried rosemary, butter, and salt. Then place on the beef fillet: grated celery root, sliced bacon, nuts, and chopped garlic. Roll the beefsteak and cover it with olive oil. Secure the meat with the help of toothpicks.

Put it on the tray and add ½ cup of water. Cook the meat in the preheated oven at 365F for 40 minutes. Meanwhile, prepare the sticky sauce: mix erythritol, lemon juice, 4 tablespoons of water, and butter. Preheat the mixture until it starts to boil. Then add the tomato sauce and beat well. Bring the sauce to a boil and remove from heat. When the beef tenderloin is cooked, remove it from the oven and sprinkle with plenty of cooked sticky sauce. Cut the meatloaf and sprinkle with the remaining sauce.

Black curry quinoa and sweet potatoes

Beans, quinoa, and sweet potatoes combine to provide a healthy and abundant portion of a meatless protein that is rewarding. You can prepare quinoa in the microwave. Follow the instructions on the package to get a cup. (250 calories per serving)

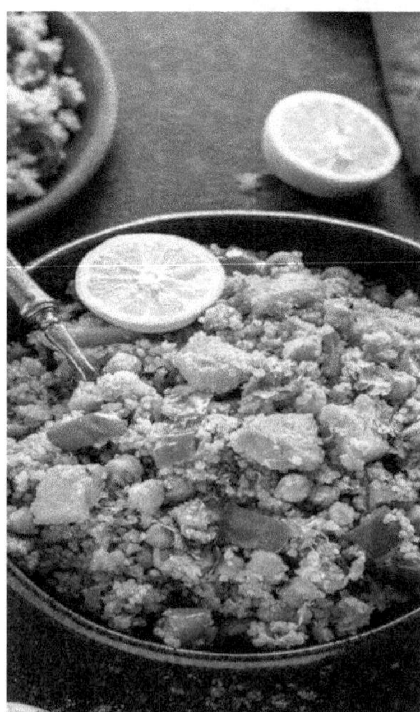

Ingredients:

- 1/2 cup quinoa.
- 1 cup of water.

- 1/2 cup sweet potato, peeled and diced (approximately 1 bit).
- 1/2 teaspoon of olive oil.
- 1/2 teaspoon dried rosemary.
- 1 cup canned black beans, drained.
- 1 teaspoon of soft curry powder.
- 2 tablespoons chopped fresh parsley.

Instructions:

Rinse quinoa under cold running water in a large mesh sieve. Drain very well and dry them on paper towels. In a small saucepan, toast the quinoa for 2 minutes over medium heat, stirring regularly. Add water and increase heat until the water boils. Cover, reduce heat and cook for 15 minutes, or until quinoa is full, and the germ forms small spirals on each grain. Remove from heat and cover to keep warm. In a small bowl, mix the sweet potato with the olive oil and rosemary. Transfer to a medium skillet over medium-high heat. Saute, frequently stirring, for 6-7 minutes or until well caramelized. Add black beans and curry, reduce heat to medium heat and cook, stirring regularly, until beans are hot. To serve, place 1/2 cup of prepared quinoa on each plate and cover with half of the bean mixture. Garnish with parsley. Makes 2 servings.

Roasted Jack Pepe Sandwiches

During roasting, instead of grilling, the cheese sandwich includes many satisfactory fries and omits excess fat. These toasted cheese sandwiches add a lot of spicy flavor to each bite. (150 calories per serving)

Ingredients:

- 2 slices of low-calorie Jack Pepe cheese.
- 4 slices of whole wheat bread with reduced calories.
- 1/2 cup fresh arugula leaves.
- 4 thin slices of fresh tomato.

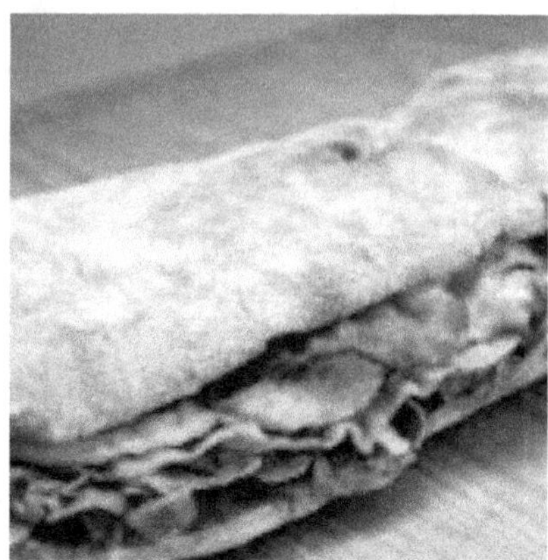

Instructions:

Preheat oven to 350 degrees F. Place 1 piece of cheese on each of the 2 slices of bread, bringing each with 2 pieces of tomato and half of arugula. Cover with the remaining pieces of bread and place the rolls on a baking sheet in the center of the oven. Toast for 4 minutes, then turn and toast for another 2 or 3 minutes or until the bread is golden, and the cheese melts. Cut each sandwich in half to serve. Makes 2 servings.

Semifreddo Peach

These frozen desserts may look good, but they are also healthier than they seem. Walnuts include omega-3 fats and fiber, as well as being crispy, and Greek yogurt has up to fourteen grams of protein per cup.

Ingredients:

- 4 medium peaches, sliced.
- 4 containers (6 ounces) of Greek vanilla yogurt.
- 1/2 cup of unsalted nuts, chopped

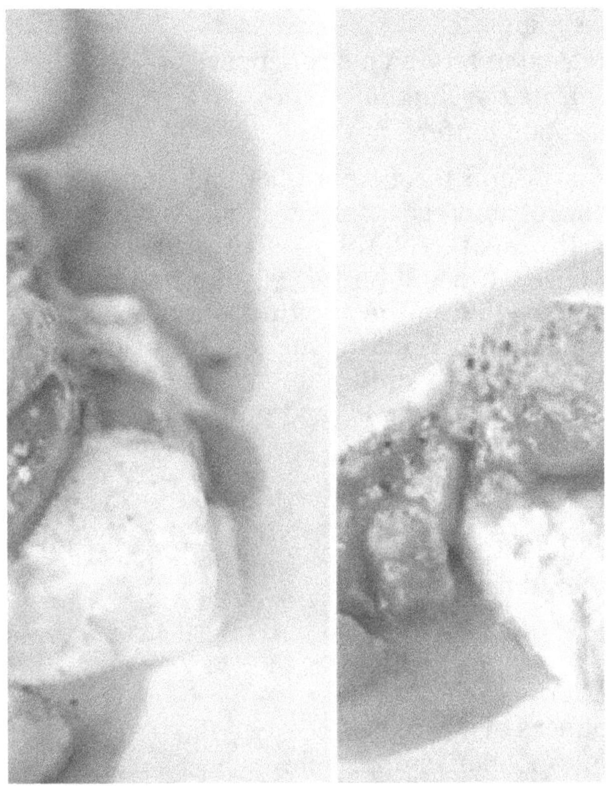

Instructions:

Divide the ingredients into 4 semi-fried desserts or start with a layer of peaches. Include a tablespoon of yogurt and then distribute the nuts. Makes 4 servings.

Fish rods

Preparation time: 10 minutes

Cooking time: 15 minutes

Servings: 6

Ingredients:

- 10 ounces of tilapia fillet
- ½ cup coconut flour
- 2 beaten eggs

- 1 teaspoon salt
- ½ teaspoon ground black pepper
- 3 oz grated parmesan
- 1 teaspoon butter

Instructions: Chop the tilapia fillet and put it in the bowl. Add coconut flour, beaten eggs, salt, ground black pepper, and grated cheese. Stir the mixture until it is homogeneous. Distribute the mold generously with the butter. Put the fish mixture in the pan and flatten it well. Cut the mixture on the bars with a knife. Preheat oven to 360F. Place the mold in the oven and cook the fish bars for 15 minutes or until the fish bars acquire the golden surface. Cool cooked food well and only then transfer it to serving dishes.

Fried cod

Preparation time: 5 minutes

Cooking time: 10 minutes

Servings : 2

Ingredients:

- 12 ounces of cod fillet
- 1 tablespoon of chopped chives
- 1 tablespoon of butter
- 1 tablespoon of coconut oil
- 1 teaspoon of chopped garlic
- 1 teaspoon of cumin seed
- 1 teaspoon coriander seeds
- 1 teaspoon salt

Instructions: Melt the butter and coconut oil in the pan. Add garlic, cumin and coriander seeds. Rub the fish fillet with salt and put it in the pan. Fry the fish for 2 minutes on each side or until it turns light brown. Transfer the cooked cod fillet to the plate and cut it into 2 portions.

Wholemeal pancakes with blueberries and nuts

These pancakes are a delicious way to start the day. Cranberries are sour, but candies and nuts add a crunchy texture to this classic of convenience.

Ingredients:

- 1/2 cup fresh blueberries
- 3/4 cup whole wheat flour

- 2 tablespoons sugar
- 1 tablespoon of baking powder
- 1/4 teaspoon salt
- 1/2 teaspoon ground nutmeg
- 1/2 teaspoon pure vanilla extract
- 1 1/4 cup low-fat milk
- 1 large beaten egg
- 1/2 cups chopped walnuts
- 1 tablespoon coconut oil, divided

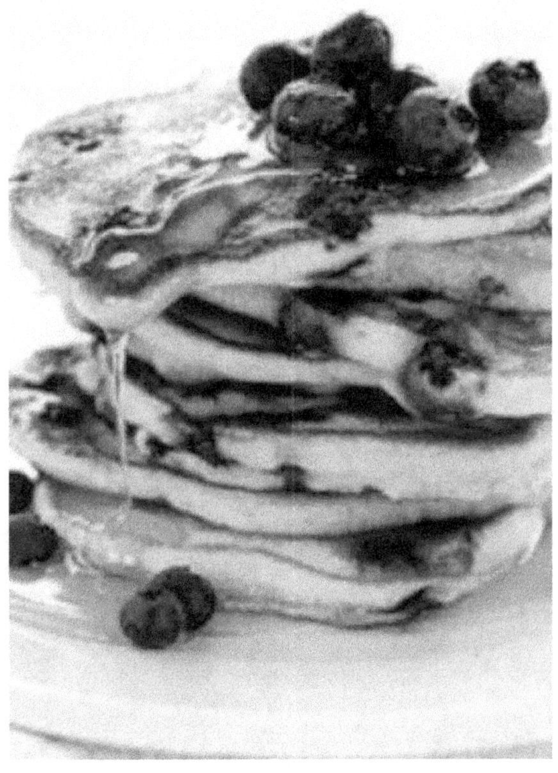

Instructions:

In a small bowl, combine the blueberries with a handful of whole wheat flour, mix well to cover. In a large bowl, add the flour, sugar, baking powder, salt, and nutmeg, stirring to mix well. Add the egg, vanilla, and milk and stir to mix; however, do not mix too much. The dough should be a bit embarrassing. Carefully add the blueberries and nuts (with flour) and set the dough aside for 10 minutes. In a large, heavy skillet, heat approximately 1/2 teaspoon of coconut oil over medium heat. Pour enough dough into the pan to make a 6-inch pancake. Cook for about 2 minutes or until the edges are bright, then turn the pancake and cook for 1 more minute. Transfer to a plate and cover while preparing the rest of the pancakes. Add extra coconut oil to the pan if necessary. To serve, put 2 pancakes on each plate and cover with hot maple syrup, honey or molasses. Makes 4 servings.

Herb and Swiss Omelette

This tortilla looks like something you would see in a restaurant. However, it only takes a few minutes to prepare. Enjoy layered flavors courtesy of moderate Swiss cheese and fresh herbs.

Ingredients:

- 2 teaspoons olive oil
- 8 large beaten eggs
- 1/2 teaspoon salt
- 1/2 teaspoon freshly ground black pepper
- 2 teaspoons chopped fresh parsley
- 2 teaspoons chopped fresh marjoram
- 1 teaspoon fresh basil chopped
- 1/2 cup shredded low-fat Swiss cheese

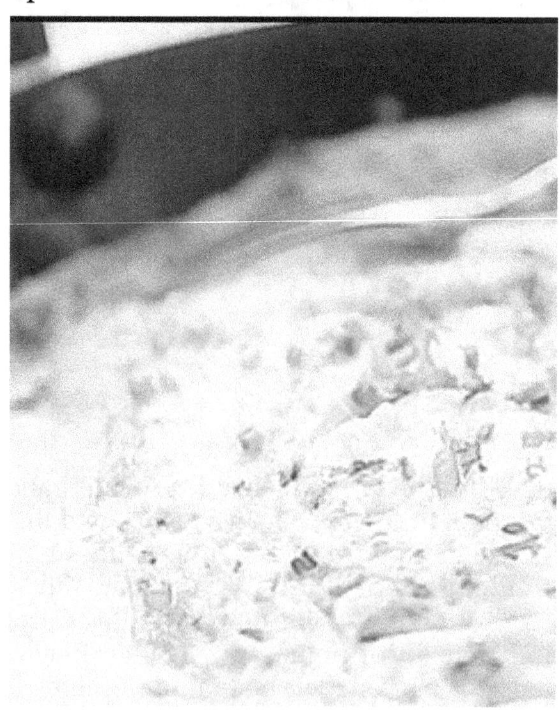

Instructions:

Preheat oven to 375 degrees F. Heat olive oil in a large oven-proof skillet over high heat. Lay the eggs in the pan, spreading them evenly. Season with salt and pepper. Remove the pan from the heat and sprinkle the marjoram, basil and parsley evenly over the eggs. Then add Swiss cheese. Place the pan in the center of the oven and cook for 18-22 minutes or until a toothpick inserted in the center is clean. To serve, cut into four pieces and serve hot. Makes 4 servings.

Zucchini Chips

Preparation time: 10 minutes

Cooking time: 12 minutes

Servings: 4

Ingredients:

- 1 finely chopped zucchini
- A pinch of sea salt
- Black pepper to taste
- 1 teaspoon dried thyme
- 1 egg
- 1 teaspoon garlic powder
- 1 cup almond flour

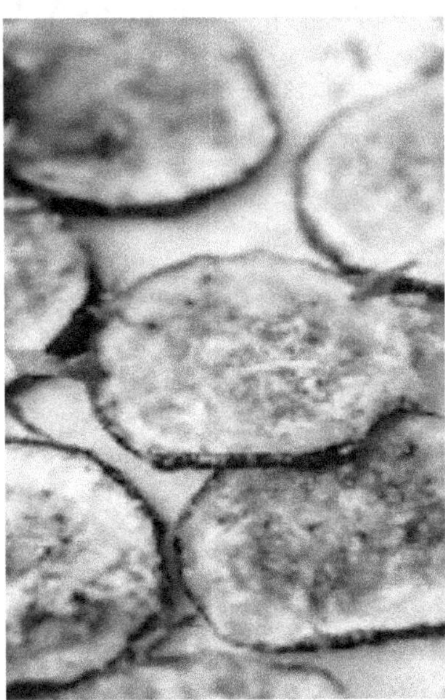

Instructions: In a bowl, beat the egg with a pinch of salt. Put the flour in another bowl and mix it with thyme, black pepper, and garlic powder. Drain the zucchini slices in the egg mixture and then in the flour. Place the french fries in a lined pan, then put them in the oven at 450° F, and cook for 6 minutes on each side. Serve the fries as a snack.

Pepper Snack

Preparation time: 5 minutes

Cooking time: 10 minutes

Servings: 24 pieces

Ingredients:

- 1/3 cup of tomatoes, chopped
- ½ cup of peppers, mixed and chopped
- 24 slices of peppers
- ½ cup of tomato sauce
- 4 ounces of almond cheese, diced
- 2 tablespoons basil, chopped
- black pepper to taste

Instructions:

Divide the slices of pepper on a muffin tray. Divide the pieces of tomato and pepper into the cups of peppers. Divide cubes, including tomato sauce, basil, and almonds, sprinkle the black pepper at the end, put the cups in the oven at 400° F, and bake for 10 minutes. Arrange the pieces of peppers in a bowl and serve. Have fun!

Holiday meatballs

Preparation time: 10 minutes

Cooking time: 40 minutes

Servings: 20

Ingredients:

- 1 kg turkey, ground
- 1 tablespoon coconut oil, melted
- 1 yellow onion, chopped

- 1 egg
- 1 cup coconut flour
- 1 teaspoon Italian dressing
- A pinch of sea salt
- Black pepper to taste
- 2 tablespoons chopped parsley

Instructions: In a bowl mix the turkey meat with half flour, a pinch of salt, black pepper, Italian seasoning, parsley, onion, egg and hot sauce and mix well. Put the rest of the flour in another bowl. Form 20 turkey meatballs and dip them in flour. Heat a pan with the oil over medium-high heat, add the meatballs and cook for 4 minutes on each side. Transfer them to paper towels to remove excess fat, put them on a plate, and serve.

Chicken fajitas

Preparation time: 10 minutes

Cooking time: 20 minutes

Servings: 4

Ingredients:

- 1 kg of tender chicken
- 1 beaten egg
- A pinch of sea salt
- 1/3 cup of coconut, unsweetened and grated
- ¼ cup of coconut flour

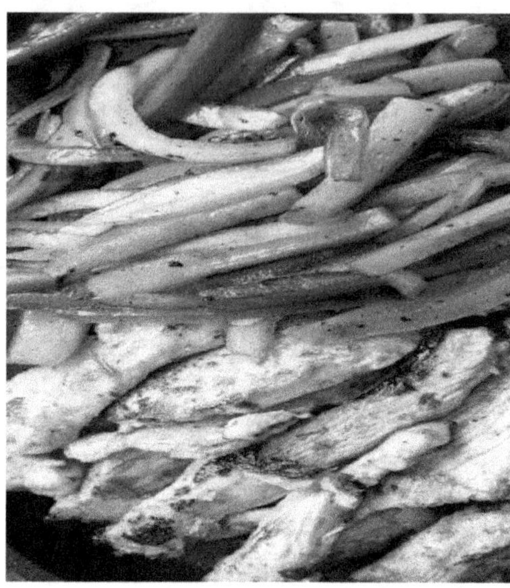

Instructions: In a bowl, mix the coconut with the coconut flour and a pinch of sea salt and mix. Put the beaten egg in another bowl. Dip the chicken pieces in the egg, then in the coconut mixture, put them in a lined pan, and bake at 350° F for 25 minutes. Serve as a snack.

Scrambled eggs with mushrooms and onions

These eggs cook quickly, but they have a flavor that will ask you to cut and enjoy it. This also makes an excellent sandwich filling. If you need breakfast on the run, an integral pita bag is an excellent option.

Ingredients:

- 1 teaspoon of olive oil.
- 1 cup sliced fresh mushrooms.
- 1/4 cup thinly sliced yellow onion
- 1 tablespoon slices of fresh tarragon.
- 1/2 cup chopped fresh parsley.
- 1/2 teaspoon salt
- 1/2 teaspoon freshly ground black pepper.
- 8 large beaten eggs.

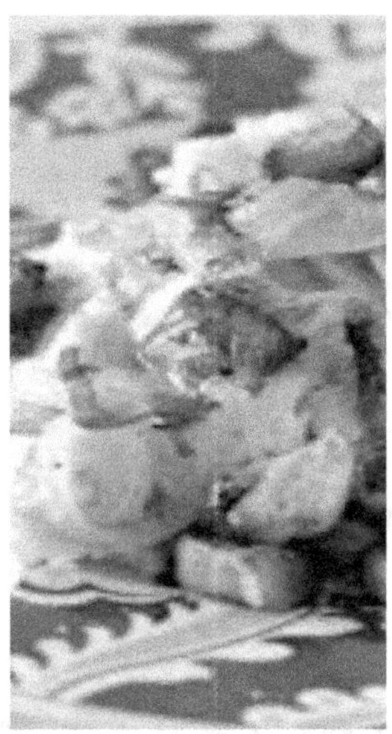

Instructions: In a large, heavy skillet, heat olive oil over medium heat. Add the mushrooms, onion, tarragon, parsley, salt, and pepper, and fry for 4 minutes, stirring occasionally. Put in the eggs and constantly stir, until they are prepared, for about 2 minutes. To serve, divide by 4 dishes. Makes 4 servings.

Grilled Fruit Salad

Fruit does not always have to be raw; In fact, toasting or roasting fresh fruit eliminates its natural sugars and increases its flavor. Duplicate the recipe and use leftovers as a side dish for chicken or seafood.

Ingredients:

- 8 slices of fresh or canned pineapple (unsweetened),
- 4 fresh nectarines or peaches, pitted and cut into 8 pieces each,
- 8 pieces (1/2 inch thick) of fresh sweet melon.
- 1 teaspoon of honey, heated for 30 seconds in the microwave
- 1/2 teaspoon of salt.

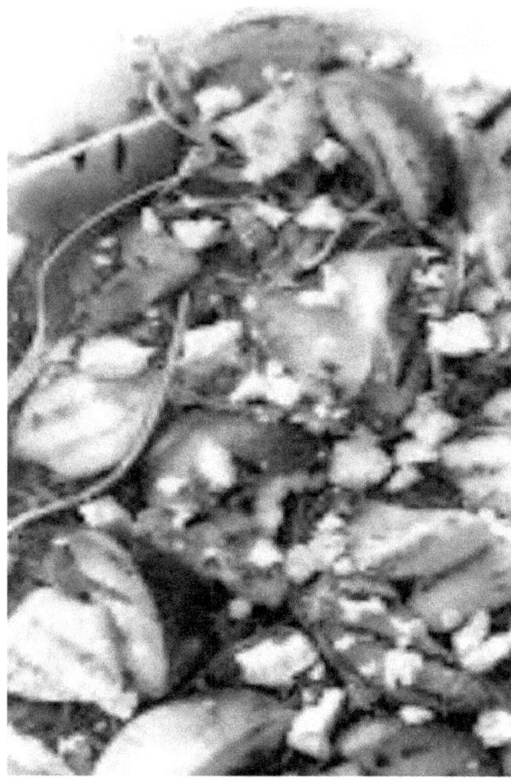

Instructions: Preheat the grill and cover a baking sheet with aluminum foil. Spread the fruit in a single layer on the baking sheet and spread with honey on both sides. Sprinkle the salt on the wire and place the pan 3 inches listed under the chicken. Cook on the grill for 3 minutes, rotate each piece of fruit, then toast for another 2 minutes, or only until the fruit is lightly browned at the edges. Put 2 pieces of pineapple, 8 slices of peach and 2 slices of melon in each of the 4 dishes and serve hot. Makes 4 servings.

Abundant hot cereal with berries.

Whole grains are not only excellent for your heart; They are also fabulous for your life. The high fiber material fills you and provides slow and steady energy for your day. The addition of berries and nuts in this dish makes it particularly abundant.

Ingredients:

- 4 cups of water.
- 1/2 teaspoon of salt
- 2 cups of whole oatmeal.

- 1/2 cup sliced walnuts.
- 2 teaspoons of flax seeds.
- 2 tablespoons honey
- 1/2 cup fresh blueberries.
- 1/2 cup of fresh raspberries
- 1 cup of low-fat milk.

Instructions: In a medium skillet, boil water over high heat and include salt. Add oatmeal, nuts, and flax seeds, then reduce heat and cover. Cook for 16 to 20 minutes or until the oatmeal reaches the preferred consistency. Divide the oatmeal between 4 deep bowls and each with 2 tablespoons of blueberries and raspberries. Add 1/4 cup of milk to each bowl and serve. Makes 4 servings.

Easy cereal bars

This dish is much better for you than any industrial granola bar, which is often loaded with high-fructose corn syrup and less healthy cereals. These bars are cooked in the blink of an eye and will be kept in an airtight container for a week, that is, if they last so long.

Ingredients:

1 teaspoon of coconut oil.

1 cup of nut pieces

1 cup of raw pumpkin seeds.

1 cup chopped nuts.

1 cup dried cranberries.

1 cup dried apricots, sliced.

1 cup unsweetened coconut flakes.

1/4 cup melted coconut oil.

1/2 cup of almond butter

1/2 cup of raw honey

1/4 teaspoon of pure vanilla extract.

1/2 teaspoon salt

1 teaspoon cinnamon powder.

Instructions:

Preheat oven to 325 degrees F. Grease a 9-by-13-inch pan with 1 teaspoon of coconut oil and set aside. In a large bowl, combine nuts, pumpkin seeds, blueberries, apricots, and coconut flakes and mix well. In a small saucepan over low heat, add melted coconut oil, almond butter, honey, vanilla, salt, and cinnamon and heat until the honey melts. Transfer the nut mixture to the pan, pushing it down to distribute evenly. Place the honey mixture evenly on top. Cook for 35 to 40 minutes or until golden brown. Allow the mixture to cool to room temperature before cutting into equal bars. Store in an airtight container for up to 1 week. Makes 1 dozen bars.

Pecans and bananas

A healthy breakfast does not always have to be hot; In fact, this is frozen. Prepare many of these tablespoons in advance and store them in the freezer. They make an exceptional gift after school. The kids will have fun!

Ingredients:

4 large and ripe bananas.

4 popsicle sticks.

1/2 cup almond butter

2 tablespoons raw honey.

3/4 cups chopped nuts.

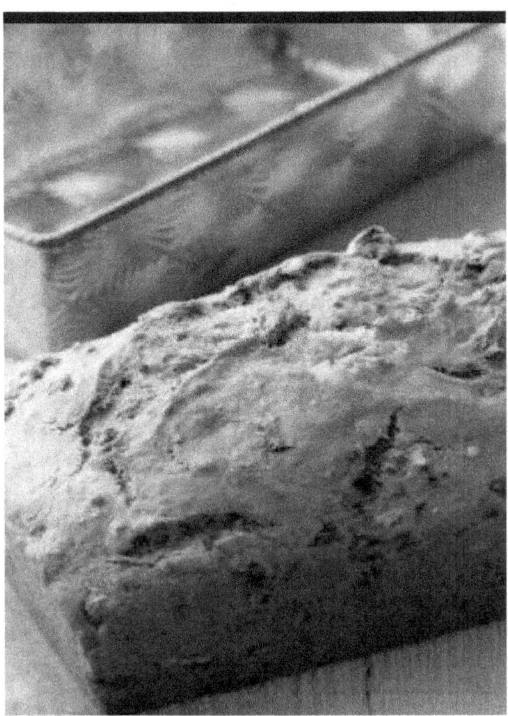

Instructions:

Peel and cut one end of each banana and insert a popsicle stick into the cut end. In a small bowl, mix the almond butter and honey and heat in the microwave for 10-15 seconds, or only until the mixture is slightly diluted. Pour onto a sheet of waxed paper or aluminum foil and distribute it with a spatula. On another piece of waxed paper or aluminum foil, spread the sliced walnuts. Line a small baking sheet or a large plate with the third piece of wax paper or foil. Initially, roll each banana in the honey mixture until it is well covered, then in the nuts until it is completely covered, gently pushing it down so that the nuts stick together. Put each whole banana on the baking sheet. When all bananas have been covered, place them in the freezer for at least 2 hours. For long-term storage, move frozen bananas into a zippered plastic bag.

Tuna and bean salad pockets

This light but hearty dish is ideal for business lunches. It loads well, and the taste improves the longer you have the opportunity to sit down, then prepare the salad at night. First, put it in a pita pocket and then in the morning lunch bag.

Ingredients:

- 4 bags of whole wheat pita.
- 1 can (6 ounces) of tuna packed in water, drained
- 1/2 can (15 ounces) of borlotti beans, rinsed and drained
- 1/4 cup chopped white onion.
- 2 tablespoons light mayonnaise.
- 1 teaspoon spicy brown mustard.
- 1/2 teaspoon of celery seeds.
- 1/2 teaspoon freshly ground black pepper.
- 1 cup sliced romaine lettuce.

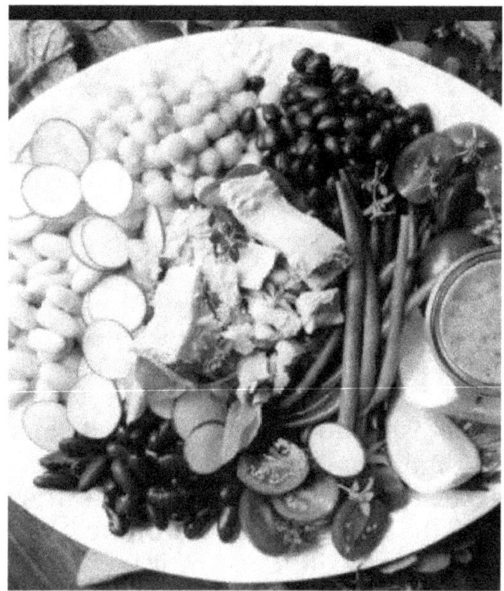

Instructions:

If the pitas are not cut, cut them so that there is an opening similar to a bag, being careful not to cut the bottom or sides. In a small bowl, add the tuna, borlotti beans, onion, mayonnaise, mustard, celery seeds and pepper, and mix well. Divide the lettuce into the pita pockets, then fill them with a quarter of a tuna salad. Makes 4 servings.

Roasted chicken breast with summer vegetables

This recipe heats up well, so prepare it for a weekend or a night and pack it in individual containers for your lunch during the week. Explore other seasonal vegetables to vary your tastes.

Ingredients:

- 4 skinless chicken breasts (4 or 5 ounces)
- 1 tablespoon olive oil
- 1 teaspoon salt, divided.
- 1/2 teaspoon freshly ground black pepper, divided
- 1/2 teaspoon turmeric powder.
- 1 medium zucchini, sliced very thin.
- 2 yellow pumpkins, thinly sliced.
- 1 medium white onion, sliced ½ inch thick
- 1 pint cherry tomatoes.
- 1 teaspoon dried parsley.
- 1 teaspoon dried oregano.

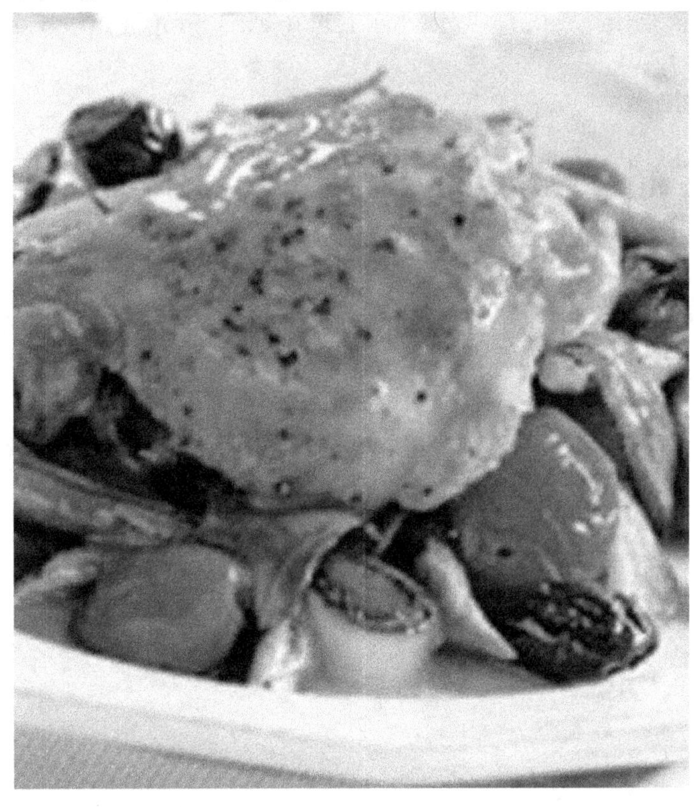

Instructions:

Preheat the oven to 400° F and cover a baking sheet with aluminum foil. Rub both sides of the chicken breast with 1 teaspoon of olive oil and season with 1/2 teaspoon of salt, 1/4 teaspoon of pepper, and turmeric. Put the chicken in the pan. In a medium bowl, add zucchini, squash, onion, and tomatoes. Include the parsley and oregano and then sprinkle with the tablespoon of olive oil. Mix the vegetables well until they are evenly distributed and distributed around the chicken breast in the pan. Bake in the center of the oven for 15 minutes, turn the chicken and mix the vegetables, then cook for another 10-12 minutes or until the chicken juices are clear. To serve, place 1 breast on each plate and cover with a quarter of the vegetables. Makes 4 servings.

Easy chicken noodle soup.

Boil the pasta one or two days in advance, and after emptying it, put it in a tightly closed bag in the refrigerator until ready to use. This little preparation work makes this soup a lunch that only takes ten minutes.

Ingredients:

- 3 cups of chicken broth.
- 1 cup of frozen green beans.
- 1 cup chopped frozen carrots.
- 1 can (6 ounces) shredded chicken, empty tubes.
- 1 teaspoon of freshly cut tarragon.
- 1 teaspoon of fresh thyme leaves.
- 1/2 teaspoon salt
- 1/4 teaspoon freshly ground black pepper.
- 1 cup of mini-shell cooked pasta.
- 1/2 cup grated Parmesan cheese.

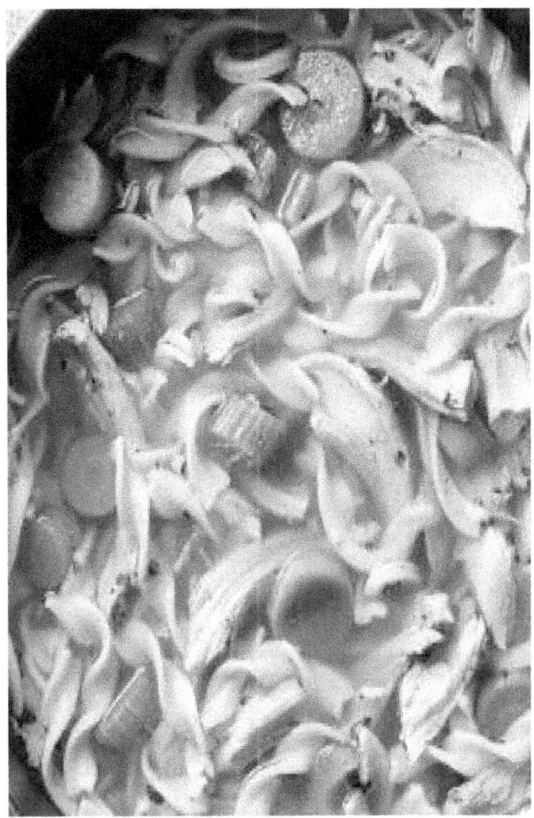

Instructions:

In a large skillet, boil the chicken stock over high heat. Add green beans and carrots and reduce heat to medium. Cover and cook for 5 minutes. Add chicken, tarragon, thyme, salt and pepper and simmer for another 4 minutes. Remove the pan from the heat and add the cooked pasta. To serve, divide between 4 bowls and add the Parmesan cheese. Makes 4 servings.

Avocado Stuffed Fish

This is an excellent light lunch, especially during the warmer months. You can prepare the filling 3 days in advance and simply assemble the food when it is ready for eating.

Ingredients:

- 1 cup cooked prawns
- 8 ounces imitated minced crabmeat
- 1 celery stalk, sliced carefully
- 1/2 red pepper, sliced
- 1/2 red onion, minced
- 2 shallots, sliced
- 2 tablespoons light mayonnaise
- 1 tablespoon of white yogurt
- 1/4 teaspoon dried mustard
- 2 teaspoons chopped fresh parsley
- 1/2 teaspoon freshly ground black pepper
- 2 avocados
- 1 teaspoon lemon juice

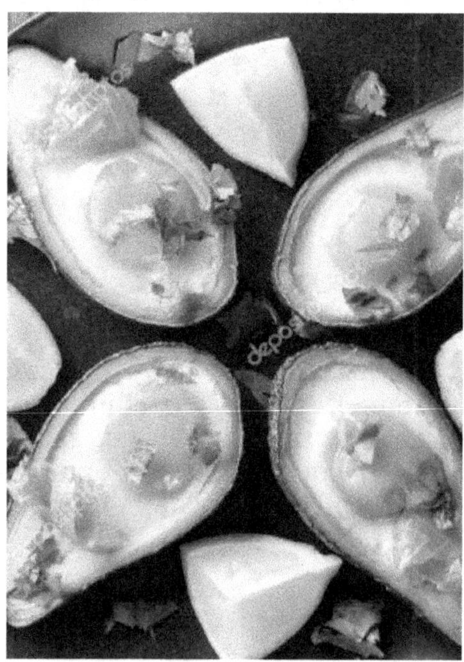

Instructions:

In a medium bowl, add prawns, crab meat, celery, pepper, onion, and chives; mix well. In a small bowl, combine mayonnaise, yogurt, dried mustard, parsley, and black pepper and mix with a fork until well mixed. Combine the mayonnaise mixture with the seafood filling until well mixed. Cut the avocados in half, remove the holes, and clean the meat with lemon juice. Fill each half of avocado with a quarter of the fish filling and serve. Makes 4 servings.

Green smoothie

Even if you don't have time for lunch, you will still have time to take many vitamins and minerals in the form of this healthy smoothie. Healthy avocado and vegetable fiber fats suggest that you will also be satisfied.

Ingredients:

- 1 medium cucumber, peeled and sliced.
- 2 cups of fresh spinach.
- 1/2 cup fresh parsley.
- 1 cup of carrot juice.
- 1/2 teaspoon of salt
- 2 drops of chili sauce.
- 1/2 chopped avocado.

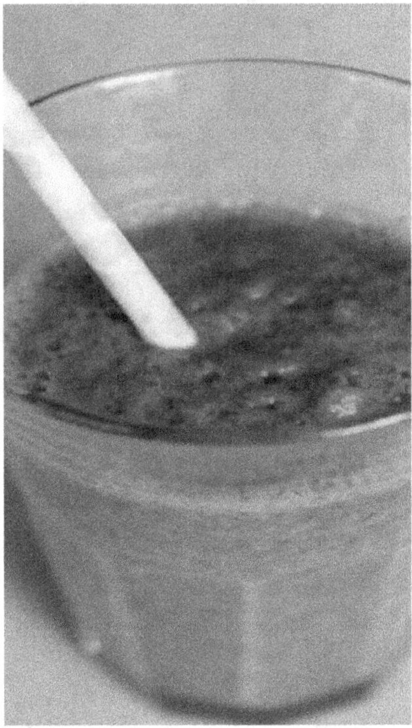

Instructions:

Integrate cucumber, spinach, parsley, carrot juice, salt, and hot sauce in a blender and mix until smooth. Add the avocado and blend at medium speed until smooth. Serve immediately. Makes 4 servings.

Toasted ham, swiss and arugula sandwiches

This toasted sandwich omits the typical ham and fatty roasted cheese and includes items that are much more crunchy. Served with a bowl of soup or a light salad, this is a delicious and healthy meal of one hour for lunch.

Ingredients:

- 8 slices of reduced calorie wholemeal bread
- 2 teaspoons of Dijon mustard.
- 1 pound (about 16 slices) of very thin sliced lean ham
- 8 pieces of low-fat Swiss cheese.
- 1 cup fresh arugula

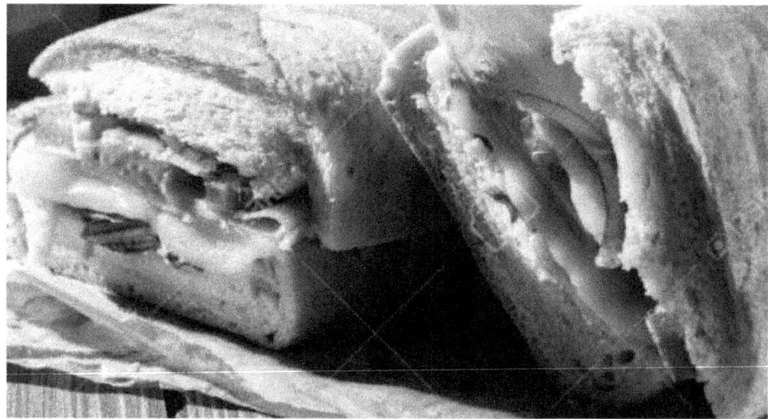

Instructions:

Preheat oven to 350 degrees F. Distribute 4 pieces of bread with Dijon mustard and cover with about 4 pieces of ham and 2 slices of cheese. Cover each with 1/4 cup arugula and place the bread pieces in the sandwiches. Bake in the center of the oven for 5 minutes, turn around and then cook for another 3 minutes or until the bread is browned and the cheese melts. Cut each sandwich in half and serve hot. Makes 4 servings.

Fast and light white bean chili

This chili takes little time (and just a pan) to prepare and tastes even better the next day. It also freezes well, then creates a double batch to divide and store in the freezer for the busiest days.

Ingredients:

- 1 teaspoon of olive oil.
- 1 kg of freshly ground turkey breast.
- 1 teaspoon of chili powder.
- 1 teaspoon of salt.
- 1/2 teaspoon freshly ground black pepper.
- 1/2 teaspoon ground cumin.
- 1 cup chopped white onion.
- 2 tablespoons chopped fresh cilantro.
- 2 cans (15 ounces) of excellent non-fatty beans
- 2 cups of chicken broth.

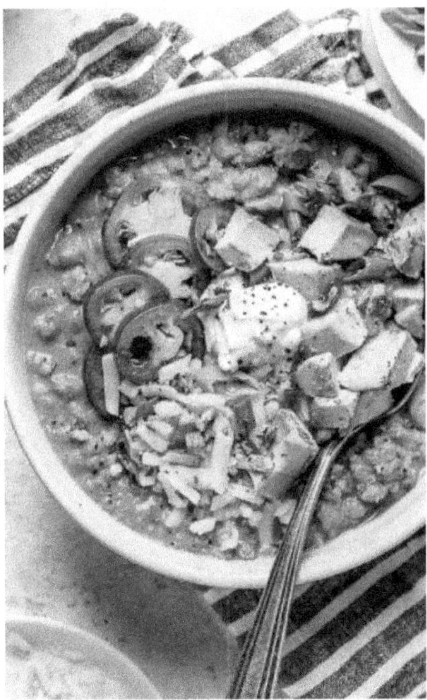

Instructions:

In a moderately heavy skillet, heat the olive oil over medium-high heat. Add turkey, chili powder, cumin, salt and pepper. Fry for 7 to 8 minutes, usually cut with a spatula, until the turkey is well cooked. Add the onion and fry for 1 more minute before including coriander, beans with liquid and chicken broth. Bring to a boil, then reduce the heat to low and simmer for 15 minutes. Divide between 4 deep plates and serve hot. Makes 4 servings.

Scrambled vegetable market

There is nothing wrong with breakfast for lunch. This meal is formulated in minutes and will keep you active all day.

Ingredients:

- 1 teaspoon of olive oil.
- 1/2 diced pepper.
- 1/2 cup chopped white onion
- 1 cup sliced fresh mushrooms.
- 1/2 teaspoon salt
- 1/4 teaspoon freshly ground black pepper.
- 8 large beaten eggs.

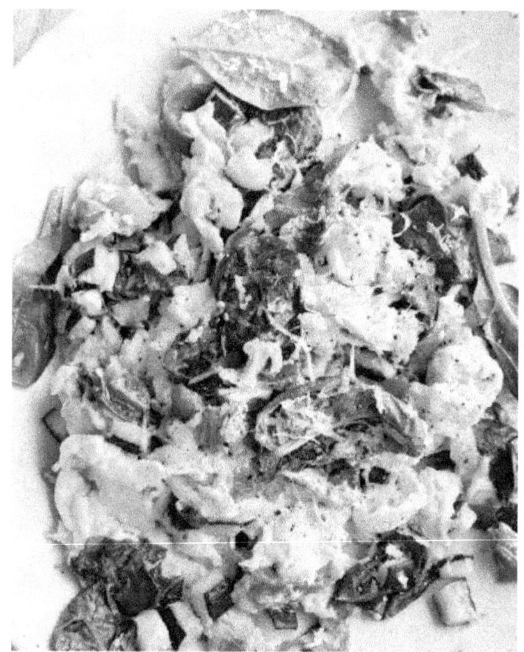

Instructions:

In a large, heavy skillet, heat the olive oil over medium heat. Add the pepper, onion, mushrooms, salt, and pepper and fry for 5 minutes, stirring frequently. Put the eggs on everything and keep stirring for about 3 minutes or until the eggs are ready. Divide between 4 dishes and serve hot. Makes 4 servings.

Chicken breast with orange spices.

This recipe offers speed and flavor. It is an excellent dish to work on the most demanding nights. Served with a green salad and some quinoa or brown rice, it is light but a pleasant meal.

Ingredients:

- 1 teaspoon of olive oil.
- 4 skinless chicken breasts (4 to 5 ounces).
- 1 teaspoon of paprika.
- 1/2 teaspoon salt
- 1/4 teaspoon freshly ground black pepper.
- 1 teaspoon sliced fresh thyme.
- 1 teaspoon of fresh sliced rosemary.
- 1 tablespoon unsweetened orange juice concentrate
- 2 tablespoons chopped fresh parsley.

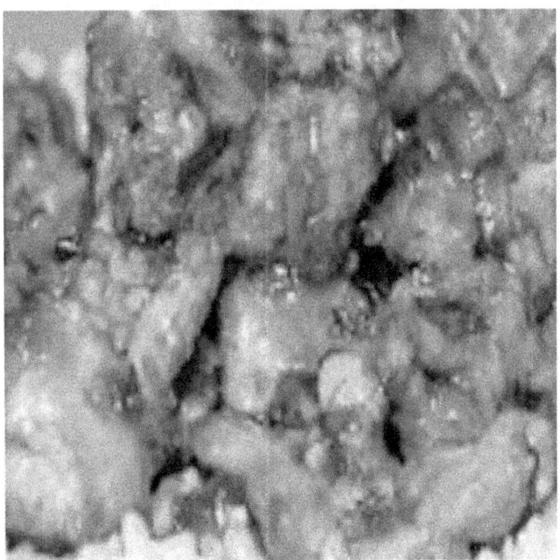

Instructions:

Preheat the oven to 400° F and cover a baking sheet with aluminum foil. Distribute olive oil on the foil. Place the chicken breasts on the foil, turn them to cover them with oil and season with paprika, salt, thyme, pepper, and rosemary. Cook for 15 minutes, then turn the chicken and spread with the orange juice concentrate. Cook for another 15-20 minutes or until the chicken juices are clear. Garnish with parsley before serving. Makes 4 servings.

Grilled shrimp and black beans salad

This dish is fantastic to use when you have a business dinner. No one will think it has low calories!

Ingredients:

- 1 teaspoon of lime zest (approximately 1/2 lime).
- 1/4 cup freshly squeezed lime juice.
- 3 tablespoons olive oil.
- 2 tablespoons sliced fresh basil.
- 2 tablespoons sliced fresh oregano.
- 1 teaspoon freshly ground black pepper.
- 1/2 teaspoon of salt
- 2 cans (15 ounces) of black beans, rinsed and drained
- 1 cup diced tomatoes.
- 1 cup diced green pepper.
- 1/2 cup chopped green onion.
- 24 large raw shrimp (21-25 counts), bare and undisclosed

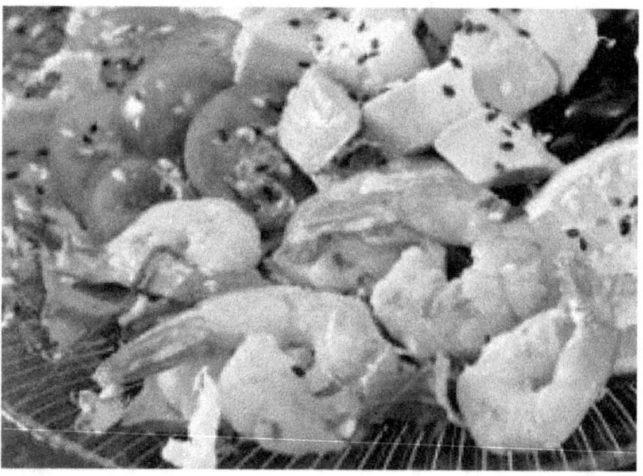

Instructions:

In a medium bowl, combine lemon juice, olive oil, basil, oregano, and pepper and mix well. Measure 2 tablespoons in a small bowl and set aside. Add salt, black beans, tomatoes, peppers, and onions in a medium bowl and mix well.

Put in the refrigerator until ready to serve. Preheat a flat grill over medium-high heat. As soon as it is hot, roast the prawns and sprinkle with the reserved lime juice mixture. Cook for 3 minutes on one side, then turn, spray again and cook for another 3 minutes. To serve, place a quarter of the bean salad on each plate and cover with 6 hot prawns. Makes 4 servings.